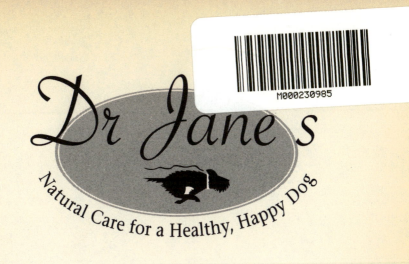

Dr Jane's

Natural Care for a Healthy, Happy Dog

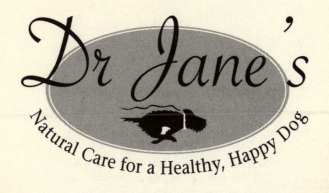

Dr Jane's

Natural Care for a Healthy, Happy Dog

JANE R. BICKS, D.V.M.

A PERIGEE BOOK

A Perigee Book
Published by The Berkley Publishing Group
A member of Penguin Putnam Inc.
375 Hudson Street
New York, New York 10014

First edition: March 1999

Published simultaneously in Canada.

The Penguin Putnam Inc. World Wide Web site address is
http://www.penguinputnam.com

Library of Congress Cataloging-in-Publication Data

Bicks, Jane R.
    [Natural care for a healthy, happy dog]
    Dr. Jane's natural care for a healthy, happy dog / Jane R. Bicks.
— 1st ed.
        p.   cm.
    "A Perigee book."
    ISBN 0-399-52482-7
    1. Dogs—Nutrition.   2. Dogs—Food.   3. Dogs—Health.
    I. Title.   II. Title: Doctor Jane's natural care for a healthy, happy dog.
    III. Title: Natural care for a healthy, happy dog.
SF427.4.B535   1999
636.7'085—dc21   98-46936
                                                                    CIP

Printed in the United States of America

10   9   8   7   6   5   4   3   2   1

Contents

Acknowledgments

It's impossible to thank every person and animal responsible for the motivation, guidance, assistance and understanding that sustained me through the years I spent writing this book. Even though I sat down to write the manuscript in 1996, the evolution of the book occurred over a span of twenty years, from the early days of veterinary school through the decades of practicing holistic veterinary medicine.

There are several people and animals who stand apart from the rest, and to them, I owe a special debt of gratitude. First is Perlane, my loyal companion in vet school who served as the nutritional model for the development of many of my remedies.

Thanks to Linda and Kevin House for the loan of Smokey for the cover photograph.

I owe a great deal of thanks and love to my husband James Rapp for his encouragement and willingness to do the housework that I was forced to neglect. With over thirteen animals, all with their own special diets of natural supplements and herbs (naturally!), this is no small task.

Finally, I must thank Michael Lutfy, my editor, for his patience and editorial guidance.

Introduction:
How Healthy Is Your Dog?

REDEFINING CANINE HEALTH

On the first day I arrived at veterinary school in Italy, a stray dog decided that I would make a suitable parent, and followed me home. I decided to name him Perlane. Brown and white, and very thin, he refused to leave my doorstep after a meal of milk, bread, and honey. I would have fed him dog food, but it was not readily available, so I had to cook his meals, morning and evening. Although still a fledgling student, I could tell this little dog was not in the best of health.

I began experimenting with new ingredients in his diet, depending on which ailments I wanted to cure at the time. It was truly a case study on the effect of nutrition on a dog's overall health and behavior. His flaky skin and dull, brittle coat, which always seemed to shed, immediately responded to the daily addition of 1 tablespoon of olive oil and one egg. His bad breath became bearable once I added fresh parsley and chopped mint to his dinner. His limp, possibly from an old injury, improved with fresh alfalfa, yucca, and cod liver oil. The townsfolk were so impressed with healthy-looking Perlane that many started to bring their problem dogs to me for nutritional, herbal consultations. By the time I had graduated, many Italian dogs owed their good health to my nutritional concoctions.

Perlane, meanwhile, became an example of a canine at its finest. Daily exercise, excellent nutrition, and love would have allowed him to reach a ripe old age if he hadn't been hit by a truck during my last year of veterinary school. He was the motivating force that directed me toward a lifelong study of nutrition and herbs. I will never forget his devoted love for me. My holistic treatment of dogs changed my definition of what a *healthy* dog should be. To say simply that a dog was not sick did not mean it was in the best of health. My expectations had increased. Change in food, exercise programs, nutritional supplements, and herbs were making a big difference in the dogs! Pain and stiffness, dry skin and coat, or lying around like the typical human couch potato was no longer the norm for my middle-aged and senior dogs. I could no longer pronounce a dog healthy based only on the evaluation I had learned in school. I had to develop a new method of evaluating the health status of a dog.

Changing foods to suit the dog and its problem helps, but through the years I have found that careful selection and use of supplements, combined with a good diet, is the real problem eliminator. I would get so exasperated treating puppy diseases—such as pimples inside their thighs, ringworm, or mange—because any specific treatment I prescribed would be temporary. They would get cured, but inevitably they came back with a second dose of illness. Why didn't all puppies succumb to these illnesses? Was the cause truly physiological, and the only cure truly pharmaceutical? What were these sick puppies lacking that the healthy ones had? What if they were fed a highly nutritious food, had herbs selected for their immune stimulation added to their diet, and were given ample sunlight and exercise? While many dog owners seemed to prefer conventional therapies because of their rapid effectiveness and their elimination of symptoms, I began to see disease differently and to rethink my approach. I learned that a dog's body is all connected, and that treating only one portion—the part that is not well—is but a Band-Aid instead of a long-term solution.

Where once I would have given steroid injections for seasonal skin disease, I now questioned the use of a substance that has side effects such as diabetes and liver disease. Again, I thought that there had to be a reason why certain dogs suffered and other dogs did not. I found that specific supplement regimes combined with the correct diet (low in allergic components, without dyes, preservatives, or sugar) could be as effective as conventional therapy. It could help to eliminate the terrible scratching and biting that drives owners to accept the side effects of conventional therapy. Omega-3 fatty acids coupled with specific antioxidants, combined with zinc, B vitamins, and bee pollen, became my successful approach to eliminating seasonal skin allergies, including flea bite allergy.

Eventually, I was able to treat animals holistically, sometimes with pharmaceuticals and sometimes without. And now, I want to share my holistic nutritional approach with you and your dog. I've tried to organize this book to make it as user-friendly as possible. Chapter 1 gives you the basics of the nutritional needs of a dog, and what goes into dog food. Chapter 2 is a rundown on the proper way to feed dogs. Chapter 3 is on supplementing to make a healthy dog healthier, or for a specific purpose, such as for a pregnant mom or a puppy.

In chapter 4, I've outlined some general and specific health and behavior problems that can be helped with nutritional aids, such as supplements and diet changes. I caution you to administer these aids only after your vet has examined your dog and approved these suggestions.

I've devoted chapter 5 to a problem many of us face with senior or neutered dogs: obesity. Obesity is just as much a health concern for dogs as it is for humans (perhaps more so). Included in this chapter is a specific weekly weight loss diet that can be repeated until the desired weight goal is reached.

In chapter 6, I've given you a brief rundown on the diet and nutritional needs of specific breeds. I used the registry of the American Kennel Club as a guideline. If you have a crossbred dog, and many of us do, go with whatever breed is dominant.

In chapter 7, I've collected the most frequently asked questions (the hip term is FAQs) into one section. If you have a question about your dog's diet and nutrition, check here first: you'll most likely find the answer.

In the appendixes you'll find reference material on vitamins, herbs, and natural supplements; a collection of recipes; and a problem/solution quick reference guide. All of these areas are frequently referenced throughout the book, so you'll become familiar with them, I'm sure.

The first step toward making sure your dog is as healthy as he can be, is to evaluate his health by using my Quality Health Checkup. Chances are that while you thought your dog was in perfect health, you will see that there is room for improvement. This book will give you the knowledge to optimize your dog's health. It doesn't matter if you have puppy or a 20-year-old dog, my diet suggestions will give your pet what it needs to be healthier and happier than before. You will see, firsthand, just how important nutrition is for a dog.

DR. JANE'S QUALITY HEALTH CHECK UP

Before you can decide which nutritional approach to take for your dog, you need to determine the state of his health. The following is a general physical you can give your dog at home.

1. Have you noticed changes in your dog's attitude or behavior, such as lethargy, restlessness, loss of appetite, trouble getting up, aggression?

2. Does the coat look dull, dry, brittle, sparse, greasy? It should be shiny, full, and healthy-looking

3. Do you see dandruff?

4. Is the skin dry or oily? Take your finger and feel at the top of the shoulders and at the rump. Normal skin should leave a slight film on your finger.

5. Is he biting and scratching himself? Is the skin irritated or sore?

6. Does your dog have an odor?

7. Are his whiskers short and broken? They should be long and full.

8. Is there a dark discharge from his eyes? (Watery, colorless discharge is common to many breeds.)

9. Are his ears tender to the touch, odorous, red, and inflamed? Normal ears should be healthy pink, without an odor.

10. Does his breath smell?

11. When you look at his teeth and gums, do you see swelling at the gum line, with or without tartar? A healthy mouth should contain white or slightly discolored teeth with pleasingly pink, healthy-looking gums.

12. When you touch the breastbone and thigh areas, are they flaccid? A well-exercised dog should have firm muscles.

13. Are your dog's ribs too prominent or simply not detectable? When you run your hands along his ribs, there should not be more than a pinch of fat and muscle over them.

14. Do you feel or see any sores or lumps as you move your hand over your dog's body, from head to tail, left side, right side, underside, and under the tail? Is the anal area red or swollen?

15. Does your dog have any fleas or ticks? If you stand your dog on a light colored towel or sheet and mess up his coat, is flea dirt or eggs (black or red specks) visible?

16. Are the pads of the feet cracked, brittle, or dry?

If you answered "yes" to any of the above, your dog may have a condition that can be alleviated with some changes in his diet, or at the very least, his general health can be improved to a higher standard. These are some of the problems that can be alleviated with the guidelines in this book. There are many supplements, herbs, and foods that will benefit your dog and will change your definition of what a healthy dog truly is.

CHAPTER ONE

Nutritional ABCs: Your Dog Is What You Feed Him

My interest in nutrition and natural remedies intensified during my first year as a veterinarian. At the time, our practice had contracts with several K9 agencies that bred guide, police, and guard dogs. Some of these dogs, although middle-aged and seniors, were in excellent health, with tight muscles, streamlined bodies, alert attitudes, shiny coats, and healthy skin. This was in direct contrast to many of the house pets I was more accustomed to examining. Although medically healthy in the physical sense, they were nowhere near as prime as these dogs, even of the same breed. What was it that made such a difference?

Second, we had a client who had three Doberman guard dogs. These dogs were magnificent, with sleek, shiny coats and well-formed muscles, and they were very alert and attentive to their owner. When I remarked on their excellent condition, he confided to me that he exercised them twice a day, fed them an alternative professional food, added a vegetable enzyme, gave them brewer's yeast and garlic treats, and washed them every two weeks.

That's when I began to evaluate foods, restudying my biochemistry, physiology, and all the technical information required to learn the science of nutrition. Which nutritional components were responsible for the youthful appearance of these working dogs? Were there really differences between dog foods?

Visits to slaughterhouses, dog food manufacturing facilities, and nutritional laboratories made it uncomfortably obvious that veterinary education had neglected a primary element in the health of the dog—its food.

Therefore, the first step on the road to a healthier, happier dog is to have a basic understanding of the basic nutritional components your dog needs to be healthy. Although the foundation of this nutrition is similar to that of humans—proteins, carbs, and fats—there are many obvious differences.

NUTRITIONAL DIFFERENCES BETWEEN DOGS AND HUMANS

Most of us consider our dogs to be members of the family, which makes it easy to forget that they have different dietary needs than we do. Few can resist a dog begging for table scraps, especially if it is a puppy. But no matter how human your dog behaves, whether it wakes you up with a wet kiss, expresses opinions about your friends, or cons you into giving up your side of the bed, its digestive system and metabolism are uniquely canine. Some specific differences are the following:

• Amino acid requirements, and thus protein requirements, are different for dogs than for humans. Human adults require 8 essential amino acids, and babies need 9, while adult dogs require 9 amino acids, and puppies need 10.

• While vitamin C is considered an essential vitamin in humans because we can't make it and must have it, it's not considered essential for dogs. They form vitamin C in their liver.

• Humans need to monitor their cholesterol levels, which generally rise in proportion to the amount of fat or meat in the diet. However, although a dog's cholesterol levels can become abnormally elevated, a meal high in saturated fats is just what they need.

• Dogs must have meat in their diet to be in optimum health. A dog's sharp canine teeth are evidence of their need to tear apart raw meat, and thus their requirement for meat. Humans, on the other hand, can eat a vegetarian diet with high grain, and maintain optimum health.

• Dogs can't handle as much cereal as humans. One reason is that humans and dogs differ in the amount of enzymes they make that are needed to break down carbohydrates. Dogs have about 80% less enzymes to break down carbohydrates than people do.

• Dog's can't handle large amounts of fiber, while humans can. When dogs are fed large quantities of fiber, it can result in constipation, excessive stool output, decreased nutrient digestion, and poor visual appearance.

• Since a dog's sense of smell is so much more sensitive than a person's a dog is less likely to eat spoiled or rancid food than we are.

• A puppy has a greater need to drink the mother's first milk (colostrum) than does a newborn child. Colostrum delivers immunity to newborns, as does the placenta. A child gets a great deal of immunity from the placenta, while a puppy gets less; thus the more important colostrum is to a puppy.

• A dog's milk contains different nutrients than a human's milk; thus a puppy can't be fed a baby formula.

• A newborn puppy requires more iron and copper than a human infant does.

• A human athlete will "carbohydrate load" before an event, while a dog athlete (sled dog) will be given high quantities of fat just before and during the event.

• A baby can begin solid food at four months, while a puppy can begin as early as six weeks.

• The gestation period for humans is nine months, while a dog's is two months. That means that a human's nutritional pregnancy demands last way longer than a dog's.

• While chocolate can have negative effects on dogs and humans, they are different. Excessive chocolate eating can make a human fat and, because of the caffeine, nervous. Chocolate, even in small amounts, can kill a dog.

Most nutritionists agree that a human diet should not contain more than 15% protein. While the protein requirement in dog food depends on the amount of fat, amino acids, and other nutrients in the food, a minimum of 18% protein is a safe requirement for an adult food. However, as with humans, a dog's nutrition is based upon adequate intake of three main nutrients: protein, carbohydrates, and fat.

PROTEIN

Protein is the foremost dietary structural material for all mammals, including dogs. It is essentially a combination of amino acids—building blocks that form thousands of different proteins (which perform specific functions). Every different amino acid configuration corresponds to a different protein, including enzymes, hormones, genes, red blood cells, hair, skin, bone, and muscle. The nine essential amino acids an adult dog must obtain from food are isoleucine, leucine, lysine, phenylalanine, threonine, valine, histidine, methionine, and tryptophan. Puppies require an additional essential amino acid, arginine.

If you've determined that your dog needs additional protein, the first thing you have to look at is the food you're feeding him, which is covered later in this chapter. Although I always recommend that you change to a food containing high-quality protein before you start supplementing, giving your dog treats such as dried liver or brewer's yeast is permissible. The important information you need is the type of protein contained in the food. While a leather shoe may contain 100% protein, most of it is unusable protein. The amount of usable protein is usually expressed in terms of biological value. Foods containing many cereal proteins (wheat, corn, barley) have little biological value, while muscle meats eggs, and organ meats such as liver have a high biological value.

The most common reasons people supplement protein beyond the minimal daily requirements is to improve skin and coat, general body composition, to help with pregnancy or lactation, and to help puppies grow. Feeding a professional alternative dog food, which is covered on page 23, with the addition of a protein treat can turn a dull, brittle, highly shedding coat into silk. This is why many breeders add eggs or brewer's yeast to their dog's food. Both are protein rich, while brewer's yeast also includes a wide array of B vitamins and minerals known as coat enhancers. A shiny coat generally indicates a healthy mom and puppies.

Benefits

• Helps growth, maintenance, and repair of all animal tissue: heart, lungs, liver, etc.

• Promotes and sustains a high-powered immune system

• Essential for a healthy brain, without which a dog can't be trained

• Promotes healthy hair, nails, and whiskers, all of which contain over 95% protein

• Promotes a healthy skeletal system: muscles, bones, tendons and ligaments

Minimum Requirements

Although a nutritionist would never measure protein quantity by looking at the percentage of protein on a label, when you look at a bag of average-quality dry food that is "complete and balanced," 18% is a safe minimum for an adult dog and 22% for a puppy. A working dog's requirement will vary depending upon its work, generally between 28% and 32%. Protein percentage on a dog food label is not an accurate measure of protein quantity, since it depends on all the other nutrients in the food. "Complete and balanced" ensures adequate protein quality and quantity as determined by the amino acids and other nutrients in the food. The average-sized dog needs 2.4 grams of protein per pound every day.

Sources

Lean muscle meat (beef, lamb, turkey, chicken), fish (cooked), egg, organ meats (kidney, liver), whole milk (casein), torula or brewer's yeast, bee pollen, wheat germ, soy, corn gluten, and wheat gluten are all sources of protein.

Deficiency Symptoms

Abdominal distention (swollen belly), hair loss, lethargy, dry, brittle hair, whiskers and nails, poor muscle development, and recurrent infections (weakened immune system) are all possible symptoms of a protein-deficient diet.

CARBOHYDRATES

Carbohydrates are nutrients derived from plants. They include starches, sugars, cereals, and plant fibers. Corn, wheat, and soy contain protein that is often used in dog food. They also serve as a back-up source of energy.

Dietary fiber is plant material made up of carbohydrates. Although dogs cannot digest it directly, it is very important for your dog. When selecting a dry dog food, be sure that it includes a moderate fermentable fiber to keep those intestinal cells healthy. Fruits or vegetables can be added to any food as a good source. If you are looking for a fiber-filled breakfast treat, you can't go wrong with oatmeal with honey, wheat germ, and lactose-reduced milk for your puppy or dog.

Rather than indulge your dog with dog biscuits (which are always fattening), feeding raw or cooked carrots, celery, or apples will provide a healthy intestinal treat without calories! Sudden changes in carbohydrate type or quantity can cause loose stool or diarrhea. While most dogs tolerate well-cooked carbohydrates, wheat can be a problem for some breeds, especially shepherds.

Benefits of Carbs

- Provide energy
- Can be a source of protein
- Can enhance food palatability (malt, molasses, honey)
- Help maintain correct glucose levels in the body
- Glycogen is essential for muscle usage

Benefits of Fiber

• Provides necessary bulk to stimulate intestinal movement of digested food, thus preventing constipation and promoting firm stool

• Helps cleanse intestine walls of digested food residue

• Helps regulate water, mineral, taurine, and sugar absorption from the intestinal tract

• Provides the intestinal cells with nutrients (short-chain fatty acids) essential for their health

• Is used for various medical conditions, depending on its type. Fiber is classified as soluble (fermentable) and insoluble (nonfermentable). For control of diarrhea, both types can be used; soluble fibers reduce water in the stool, while insoluble fibers can slow intestinal movement. For constipation and obesity management, insoluble fiber is added to food. Use soluble fibers for intestinal health. Both insoluble and soluble fibers are useful for insulin management in diabetic dogs.

Minimum Requirements

Although dogs have no standard requirements for carbohydrates, for optimal health (especially during pregnancy and lactation) they need at least well-processed rice, corn, or wheat. Dry dog foods contain anywhere between 30% and 60% carbohydrates, while canned foods have up to 30%. An average nonworking dog does well with a diet of 36% carbohydrates. At least 1% moderately fermentable fiber is necessary for intestinal health. Most maintenance pet foods contain 3–6% fiber, and weight-loss foods can contain as much as 17% fiber.

Sources

For backup energy: well-processed corn, wheat, barley, oats, or rice. Soluble fibers: beet pulp, gum arabic and xanthan gum, pectin, fruits, beans, avocado, artichoke, vegetables. Insoluble fibers: cellulose, lignin, peanut hulls, cereal grains.

Deficiency Symptoms

Pregnant and lactating dogs have difficulty maintaining weight, healthy-looking skin, and a sense of general well-being without carbohydrates added to their diet. Chronic constipation can indicate a deficiency of fiber. High quantities of fiber can decrease nutrient absorption and thus jeopardize general health.

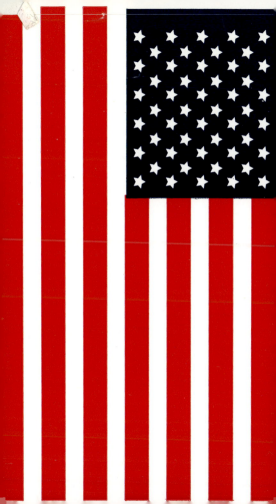

FATS

Fats are the most concentrated source of your dog's dietary energy. Fat contains approximately twice the calories of carbohydrates or protein. Oils are the liquid form of fat. Fats are composed of fatty acids. Those of prime importance for your dog are linoleic, linolenic, and arachidonic. Fortunately, dogs can synthesize the latter two, provided there is enough linoleic acid in the diet. Vegetable oils (corn, soy, peanut, safflower) are rich in linoleic acid; meat fats (tallow and lard) contain small amounts of linoleic acid and more arachidonic acid. Fish oil is rich in linolenic and arachidonic acids.

Fats form vitamins F, A, D, E, and K (fat-soluble vitamins) in the body and enable them to be utilized properly. They serve as building blocks for hormones such as estrogen, progesterone, and testosterone. Fats are important for a healthy nervous system, and are classified into the types omega-3, -6, or -9. Omega-3 fats are involved with the body's response to inflammation, swelling, redness, and itching.

In order to evaluate pet food, you need to know that two types of fat are used; soft and hard. Because soft fat melts easily, it is readily digested and extremely beneficial to your dog. Lard and chicken fat are soft. These are listed on the dog food label. If animal fat is listed on the label, the food probably contains a hard fat, such as tallow.

While the addition of a little chicken fat never hurt any dog, too much of a good thing can be bad. Large amounts of fat or oil of any type will make your dog sick, fat, and probably very oily. If you want your dog's coat to shine, add a balanced fatty acid supplement. It will contain support nutrients to make sure the fatty acids are used properly.

If fats are to be stored, preservatives (natural or chemical) must be added to them. Natural foods can contain chemical preservatives within the fat that you don't know about. The label regulations allow the manufacturer to state that its food is natural as long it isn't the one putting preservatives into the food. When a label reads "Fortified with Vitamins & Minerals," it is likely there are chemical preservatives in the food.

Benefits

- Makes food more palatable

- Supplies needed energy, especially during growth or stress

- Promotes healthy skin and coat

- Is essential for healthy nervous and immune systems

- Assists in temperature regulation, especially during the winter

- Omega-3-type fats, in combination with other nutrients, can help decrease inflammation in various parts of the body.

How Much Is Needed

• A balanced, maintenance dry dog food should contain between 5% and 13% fat, while one for performance, gestation, or lactation can contain as much as 25% fat.

• The Association of American Feed Control Officials (AAFCO) Canine Nutrient Profile recommends a minimum of 1% linoleic acid and 5% total fat for maintenance, and 8% for growth and reproduction, for dry food. This does not take into consideration the different types of fat or the individual requirements of the dog.

Sources

• Soft animal fat (chicken fat, bacon grease, or lard), butter, fish oils

• Vegetable oils like corn, soy, and safflower contain linoleic acid. These are sources of omega-6 fats. Vegetable oils like flax, primrose, and borage contain linolenic acid, sources of omega-3 fats

• Hard animal fat (tallow)

Deficiency Symptoms

• Dry skin, dandruff, dull coat, excessive itching and scratching, lethargy, reproduction problems, frequent illnesses, and cracked pads are signs of fat deficiency.

DECIPHERING DOG FOOD

No matter what vitamins, minerals, herbs, and other stuff we add to a food, it's the food that delivers most of your dog's basic nutrition. Think of your dog's food as the base of a nutritional pyramid. It supplies the scientific balance of nutrients that all dogs require, while the other levels of the pyramid are reserved for the supplements that your dog requires to be healthy and happy. Thus, whether you feed dog food with or without supplements, treats, or table scraps, you've got to select the dog food that is most appropriate for your dog. This section is designed to help you do just that.

Reading the Label

All pet foods are regulated by the American Association of Feed Control Officials, the Food and Drug Administration, the Center for Veterinary Medicine, the U.S. Department of Agriculture, and the Federal Trade Commission. There are strict regulations that require manufacturers to include certain information on the label. Although the label doesn't tell us the whole story, it certainly gives us enough to start our food investigation. Here's an example of what a typical dog food label may look like.

BRAND XYZ	(brand name)
Beef Chunk Dinner	(product Name)
For Dogs	(designator)
NET WT 23-¼ oz. (659 gms.)	(net weight statement)
Complete and Balanced	(nutrition statement)

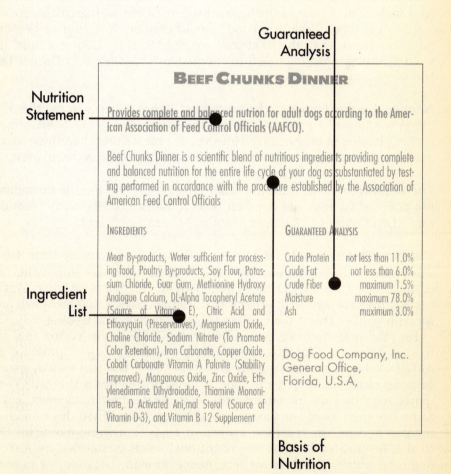

Guaranteed
Analysis

BEEF CHUNKS DINNER

Nutrition
Statement

Provides complete and balanced nutrion for adult dogs according to the American Association of Feed Control Officials (AAFCO).

Beef Chunks Dinner is a scientific blend of nutritious ingredients providing complete and balanced nutrition for the entire life cycle of your dog as substantiated by testing performed in accordance with the procedure established by the Association of American Feed Control Officials

INGREDIENTS

GUARANTEED ANALYSIS

Ingredient
List

Meat By-products, Water sufficient for processing food, Poultry By-products, Soy Flour, Potassium Chloride, Guar Gum, Methionine Hydroxy Analogue Calcium, DL-Alpha Tocopheryl Acetate (Source of Vitamin E), Citric Acid and Ethoxyquin (Preservatives), Magnesium Oxide, Choline Chloride, Sodium Nitrate (To Promote Color Retention), Iron Carbonate, Copper Oxide, Cobalt Carbonate Vitamin A Palmite (Stability Improved), Manganous Oxide, Zinc Oxide, Ethylenediamine Dihydroiodide, Thiamine Mononitrate, D Activated Ani,mal Sterol (Source of Vitamin D-3), and Vitamin B 12 Supplement

Crude Protein	not less than 11.0%
Crude Fat	not less than 6.0%
Crude Fiber	maximum 1.5%
Moisture	maximum 78.0%
Ash	maximum 3.0%

Dog Food Company, Inc.
General Office,
Florida, U.S.A,

Basis of
Nutrition

Defining the Terms

Now, let's define some of these terms on the label.

The Brand Name: The brand name is not required by law but most dog foods list it; for example, Alpo or Iams.

The Product Name: Not required by law; usually describes that particular food, e.g., beef chunks.

Using an Ingredient in the Name: Sometimes a manufacturer names its food in terms of a major ingredient: beef, chicken, or turkey. In order to do so, a minimum of 95% of the food must consist of that ingredient. For example, "Dr. Jane's Beef Dog Food" would contain 95% beef or beef by-products. However, if the food contains only 25% beef, for example, the word "Dinner" must be added to the name: "Dr. Jane's Beef Dinner Dog Food."

Naming Specific Meats in the Ingredient Panel: When you see the term "meat" or "meat by-products," that meat can be beef, pork, sheep, or goat without having to be specified. However, if a meat other than these four is used, it must be named on the label. An example would be horse meat.

The Designator: This indicates what type of dog the food is formulated for: puppies, fat dogs, old dogs, etc. Diet foods can be labeled as "Reduced Fat," "Less Calories," "Reduced Calories," "Lean," or "Light."

Nutrition Statement: This is one of the most important parts of the label. It indicates if the dog food contains all of the nutritional components recommended by the AAFCO. Some dog foods are not complete and balanced because they are used with other foods. In that case the statement will read something like "This product intended for supplemental feeding only."

Pet food manufacturers generally use two methods to ensure that the food is balanced. The first is to follow a simple "recipe" provided by AAFCO. While ingredient quality and cooking method will vary by manufacturer, rather than feed the food to dogs and perform the AAFCO-required tests, they use ingredient tables of value (recipes) that allow them to formulate their food. The food is not tested on dogs. When this numerical method is used, the nutrition statement reads something like "This dog food is formulated to meet the nutritional levels established by AAFCO dog food nutrient profiles for (pregnancy, growth, lactation, or maintenance)."

With the second method, the manufacturer follows a "recipe" and then test-feeds the food to dogs. It then evaluates the general health, stool volume, and basic blood values to determine if the recipe really delivered what it was supposed to. Those of you who enjoy cooking know how often the recipes you followed don't turn out the way they were supposed to. Of course testing is necessary! When this method is used, the nutrition statement reads something like "Animal feeding tests using AAFCO procedures substantiate that (blank) dog food provides complete and balanced nutrition for (pregnancy, growth, lactation, or maintenance)."

Some manufacturers who verify their formulation by testing will exceed certain AAFCO-suggested ingredient quantities as well as the AAFCO-required testing, performing long-term studies (kidney, liver, and heart function, bone growth) to determine the effect of their formulation in the dog. These are the ones I depend upon.

The Guaranteed Analysis: While some manufacturers will provide you with more numbers, AAFCO requires only the protein, fat, fiber, and water percentage in the food. The water percentage is important because the more water in the food, the fewer the nutrients.

The fat percentage is obviously important so you know if your dog is on a high- or low-fat diet, but equally important is the ratio of fat to protein—the closer, the better. A dry dog food with a crude protein of 30% and a crude fat of 20% is a better choice than one with a crude protein of 30% and 8% fat. Without substantial fat, the protein, no matter how good it is, simply doesn't get used efficiently. I prefer chicken or pork fat over tallow.

The protein percentage tells you how much protein is in the food, but it doesn't tell you what type of protein it is. Many cereals and other plant proteins do not have the quality that meat protein has (assuming it is good-quality meat). I like to see a meat protein as the number one ingredient, and no more than two cereals.

Ingredients: These are listed according to their quantities in the food, from most to least. The first ingredients listed are contained in larger volume than those listed much later. You've got to read the list, no matter how fine the print and how foreign it sounds. It must follow AAFCO's definitions.

DEFINING THE INGREDIENTS

The following are commonly used ingredients in most commercially available dog foods.

Meat, Chicken, Poultry, or Fish

The term "meat" indicates that you are feeding your dog the muscle meat from an animal. The meat can be beef, pork, goat, lamb, or mutton. If another type of meat is used (venison, rabbit, etc.) then it must be specifically stated. The term "chicken" implies chicken only, while the term "poultry" can include turkey or pheasant. Your carnivore dog can derive excellent protein from these ingredients, depending upon the combination and amount of fat, tendons, ligaments, and blood vessels the manufacturer uses. Generally speaking, the cleaner the muscle meat, the better.

Meat By-products: "By-products" are defined as the clean parts of slaughtered animals other than the muscle. They include the lungs, spleen, heart, kidneys, brain, liver, blood, bone, fat, stomach, and intestines. They do not include hair, horns, teeth, or hoofs. The by-products used will depend upon the level of nutrition the pet food manufacturer wants to deliver. Organs such as kidney and liver are an excellent source of protein with a high biological value, while bone, fat and intestines are less nutritious. The label doesn't have to specify the type and amount of by-products used, so you really don't know.

Meat Meal: "Meal" is produced from dehydrated animal tissue without the blood, hair, hoofs, horn, hide, or stomach. The major difference between this and "meat" is the amount of water content. Less water means more meat in concentrated form, which translates into more nutritional value. Meat meal is a good choice.

Meat and Bone Meal: This is a product from animal tissues including bone. It can't include blood, hair, hoof or horn. While it is a great source of calcium and phosphorous, its protein value can be limited.

Poultry: This is a combination of flesh and skin, with or without the bones, of chicken, turkey, or pheasant. It can't contain feathers, heads, feet, or entrails.

Poultry Meal: This is the dry product derived from the flesh and skin of chicken, pheasant, or turkey. It can't have any feathers, heads, feet, or intestines.

Poultry By-product Meal: This is defined by AAFCO as the ground, clean parts of poultry, including necks, feet, kidneys, livers, underdeveloped eggs, and intestines. Water is taken out so that the product is in dry form, and therefore concentrated. Feathers are not allowed. The quality of this meal depends upon the manufacturer, and is not indicated on the label. It can be an excellent source of protein, however.

Poultry By-products: By-products are defined by AAFCO as clean parts of carcasses of poultry such as heads, feet, livers, and kidneys. The quality depends upon the manufacturer. By-products can be an excellent source of protein.

Glandular Meal: This consists of dried liver and glands from slaughtered animals. It is a great flavor booster, and it can also serve as a protein source, thus increasing the protein percentage of the food.

Animal Digest: This consists of animal tissue that has been broken down into a liquid or powder. It is used for flavor. Liver digest contains liver, chicken digest contains chicken, etc.

Fish Meal: Fish meal consists of the clean, dried, ground tissue of the whole fish, with or without the oil. It can't contain more than 3% salt unless "fish meal" is part of the brand name.

Fish Liver and Glandular Meal: This is the dried whole viscera of the fish, with at least 50% consisting of liver and 18 mg. minimum of riboflavin.

Fish By-products: These consist of clean parts of the fish, such as head, fins, tail, skin, bones, and viscera. Nutritional value depends on the parts included.

Milk and Egg Products

These can be excellent sources of protein and are generally in the form of whole eggs, cheese, whey, casein, or dried milk protein. Whey is the liquid left after the curd and cream are separated from the milk. It can cause intestinal problems in lactose-sensitive dogs or dogs allergic to dairy products. Casein is a protein found in defatted milk. It will cause problems in dogs who are allergic to dairy products.

Vegetable Protein and Carbohydrates

These ingredients take the form of ground soybeans; soybean meal; soy, wheat, or rice flour; textured soy protein; wheat or gluten meal; ground sorghum, corn, or barley; wheat germ meal; corn, wheat, or rice flour; or oat groats (clean oats without the hull).

Fiber

Fiber may be added in the form of apple pomice; beet pulp; peanut, soybean, or rice hulls; rice bran or polishings; tomato pomace; or cellulose.

Fats

Fats are important for your dog. Animal fat can be chicken fat (very digestible) or tallow (hard fat). Chicken fat means just that. Vegetable oils can include corn, safflower, and other types. Some manufacturers name the individual oils they use.

Preservatives and Additives

Without getting too scientific, preservatives you'll likely encounter will include sodium nitrate or nitrite, which is thought to be carcinogenic; monosodium glutamate (MSG); butylated hydroxyanisole (BHA); butylated hydroxytoluene (BHT); ethyoxyquin; benzoic acid; propyl gallate; and guar gum. Additives include caramel and titanium dioxide for coloring.

Vitamins and Minerals

There will be a list of the vitamins and minerals on the label. For more information, go to Appendix A to get the lowdown on each mineral and vitamin, what it does, and the recommended amount.

COMPARING DRY AND CANNED OR SEMIMOIST FOOD LABELS

The major difference between these forms of dog food is the amount of water in them. In order to compare the gross analysis (percentage) of a dry food with a canned or a semimoist food, all you have to do is remove the 80% water from the canned food, 10% from the dry, and about 78% from the semimoist food. Now, you can compare their percentages of dry ingredients. Look at the following example and compare the protein amounts.

DR. JANE'S DRY DOG FOOD		DR. JANE'S CANNED DOG FOOD	
Protein	20%	Protein	5%
Fat	20%	Fat	6%
Fiber	10%	Fiber	1%
Moisture	10%	Moisture	80%

Canned Food Calculations

To find out how much of the canned food is dry ingredients, subtract the percent of water from 100% (100–80 = 20% dry ingredients). To find out how much protein is in the dry ingredients, divide the percentage of protein on the label by the percentage of dry ingredients: 5 divided by 20 is 25%.

Dry Food Calculations

Dr. Jane's canned dog food contains 25% protein on a dry matter basis (without the water). To find out how much of the dry food is dry ingredients, subtract the percent of water from 100% (100–10% = 90% dry ingredients). To find out how much protein is in the dry ingredients, divide the percentage of protein on the label by the percentage of dry ingredients (20 divided by 90 = 22% dry ingredients). Thus, you can be sure that this dry food does indeed contain more protein than the canned, but that is not always the case. Don't take these conversions lightly.

TYPES OF DOG FOOD

By now, you should know more than you did about the food you are feeding your dog. But dog food, as you know, comes in several different forms. Once you have compared the gross percentage of the various food types, you need to decide if you should you use canned, dry, semimoist, home-cooked, or a combination. Much of this decision depends on the specific needs of your dog. Let's list the pros and cons of each type to help you determine what might be best for your dog.

Canned Food

Some of the advantages of using canned food are the following:

• It is high in fat, and therefore more palatable than dry food.

• It contains more digestible meat proteins than most dry food.

• The food is cooked in the can, destroying potential disease-causing bacteria.

• It has a longer shelf life than dry or semimoist foods, and it requires fewer, if any, preservatives.

• You can hide Fido's medicine in it.

• It's soft and easy to chew for dogs that have lost teeth.

Some of the disadvantages are the following:

• The high water content (75–78%) means less nutrition per cup than dry food.

• It is probably the most costly way to feed your dog.

• The canning process can cause loss of nutrients.

• Many brands contain color additives, which I personally believe could be cancer-causing.

• Many manufacturers disguise soy or vegetable-textured protein so it looks like animal protein.

• It needs to be refrigerated after opening.

• It can't be left out all day because it will go bad or attract pests.

Semimoist Food

Semimoist food is defined as a soft, textured, bite-sized food that contains meat, cereal, water, and chemicals to reduce spoilage. It's a cross between dry food and canned food. It can have 15–50% water. Some advantages are the following:

- It comes in convenient, easy-to-serve pouches.

- It doesn't spoil if left out, the way canned does.

- It contains less water than canned, and therefore has more nutritional value, but still not as much as dry food.

- It is very tasty to your dog.

- It can be used as a treat.

Some of the disadvantages are the following:

- Most semimoist foods contain artificial coloring and preservatives, some of which may have the potential to cause cancer.

- It costs more than equivalent dry dog foods.

- The sugar in it can cause behavior problems. It's not recommended for hyper dogs.

- It can be high in salt.

- It can be difficult to get a dog to change from semimoist to dry food or even to canned.

Dry Food

Dry food is the most inexpensive way to feed your dog because of the low moisture content (10–12%) and the high concentration of nutrients. It can also be purchased in bulk for additional savings. Some other advantages are the following:

- Dry food doesn't require refrigeration.

- It can be left in the dish all day without spoiling.

- It can promote dental health if your dog chews.

- It generally has a better nutritional analysis than canned food because of the low water content.

- It is great for feeding pregnant or lactating dogs and puppies.

- It is great for feeding working dogs.

Some of the disadvantages are the following:

• It is susceptible to insects, mold, and fungi.

• Some supermarket brands are frequently lower in fat, and therefore less palatable than canned or semimoist food.

• Many brands contain artificial preservatives, and sometimes coloring.

• It has a shorter shelf life than canned or semimoist.

• Dry food left available all day can lead to obesity.

• Many dry foods contain primarily cereal protein rather than meat protein

Home-Cooked Food

Home-cooked food gives you a measure of control over what you are feeding you dog. Some advantages are the following:

• You can select the quality of ingredients you want, leaving out all artificial ones.

• Recipes can be tailored to your dog's palate.

• Generally it is very tasty.

A disadvantage is that recipes are frequently unbalanced and deficient in necessary nutrients

I recommend that all dogs be fed dry food, except for the senior that has lost teeth. If you have a puppy (miniature size or giant), although you may think that his little teeth require canned food, they don't. Dry puppy foods are slightly softer or have a form that makes eating easier. Leaving a measured amount of food down all day allows your puppy or dog to nibble as he requires, and can decrease destructive hungry behavior. While adult dogs who have not been brought up this way may eat the food all at one time, controlled nibbling is really the most natural method of feeding dogs, and some dogs can be converted.

For finicky dogs, dogs that require supplements or medication in their food, or anxious owners, mixing a canned food with a dry food is acceptable if the canned food is of the same brand or is not 100% nutritional, so that it does not throw off the balance.

Where to Buy Dog Food

Now that you know how to read a dog food label, and have some idea of the type you want, you need to decide where to buy it. This is a more important choice than it sounds, because the best food isn't always the most readily available. Where you buy your food is almost as critical as what you buy. I've grouped the sources for these foods into two general categories, supermarket/commercial food and alternative food. The difference in quality between the two is great. To put it plain and simple, many major-brand supermarket foods are to alternative foods as junk/fast food is to my grandmother's home cooking. The K9 agency dogs and the guard Dobermans mentioned at the beginning of this chapter were fed alternative foods, bought from veterinarians or pet supply stores, while most family pets I had been seeing that were not nearly as healthy were being fed name brands from the supermarket. The alternative dog foods generally offered a higher level of nutrition that translated into healthier looking dogs. Better-quality proteins and fats allowed the dogs to reach their full genetic potential, building muscle, long, beautiful coats, and alert minds. Breeders know the secret of nutrition power and how it can mean the difference between winning a ribbon or simply being a me-too dog.

Supermarket/Commercial Food Sources

Pet owners spend an astounding $7 billion per year for dog and cat food, and many new foods enter the market to capture a piece of it. Major-brand supermarket foods have been part of this industry for more than 40 years, offering tasty, affordable food that will deliver adequate, balanced nutrition. Because these companies advertise extensively on television and in magazines, that cost is often offset by the quality of the ingredients in the food. Ingredients may vary in quality and amount depending on the ups and downs of the commodities market. Supermarket dog foods will change quantities of ingredients depending upon price, and are thus considered "nonfixed-ingredient foods." That means the food can vary from batch to batch. A particular brand of food bought one week may have a little more corn or rice, or a different mix of chicken parts, than the same food bought another week. While this may not bother you, stressed, sick, pregnant, lactating, or food-sensitive dogs may respond to these changes with gastrointestinal problems.

Dog food ingredients are expensive, especially meats (chicken, fish, beef, poultry by-products, etc.) and good-quality fats. In order to reduce the cost of the food, many of these manufacturers use cereal proteins, such as soy, corn gluten, rice gluten, wheat, or barley, rather than meats. While these cereals can be formulated to give tested, well-balanced nutrition, the proteins and fats used rarely result in the type of health that breeders and veterinarians expect.

This is not to say that there is something wrong with the major-brand supermarket foods; it's just that their standard for what constitutes a healthy dog is often based upon different criteria—to the commercial food manufacturer, a dog with dandruff, dry or oily skin, a matted coat, and large stools is within the acceptable limits of health.

To be fair, not all supermarket manufacturers are alike. Beware of generic foods (no thrill) and any foods that say "manufactured for" rather than "by." These foods simply don't have the science and research behind them that ensure adequate nutrition. Major-brand manufacturers generally have their own research facilities, staffed with teams of scientists and veterinarians who have contributed significantly to understanding canine nutrition. Their testing far exceeds the required minimal AAFCO testing of only 26 weeks. You can be assured of nutrient balance and good quality control.

Alternative Food Sources

Shiny, long, full coats and compact, nonodorous stools are generally a result of higher-quality meat proteins and fats. Companies that are willing to invest in this higher level of nutrition need to sell their products for more, and thus place them in places where ingredients can be explained to the consumer, such as in pet shops, feed stores, health food stores, breeders' facilities, and veterinarians' offices. While many alternative foods are good, and can put supermarket foods to shame, others can be equated to generic, no-frills dog food with wholesome-sounding ingredients. I have therefore divided alternative dog foods into two categories, professional and nonprofessional.

Professional: Among the dog food manufacturers who distribute their product in alternative places, there is a group that takes optimum nutrition very seriously. Their labels read "manufactured by," and they have research facilities and scientists who produce consistently high-quality food. The ingredients are "fixed" and based on scientific data gathered through research above and beyond the simple AAFCO feeding tests. These companies are generally very involved with university studies to provide new information regarding disease and nutrition in our pets. Foods manufactured by these companies are the ones that I recommend most.

Non-Professional: These foods are sold in the same alternative markets as the professional ones. Since the dog owner expects better results from alternative dog foods than from supermarket brands, they tend to have more meat and fat than supermarket dog foods. While their quality and dependability differ from company to company, they generally contain lower-quality ingredients or more cereals than their professional counterparts. Minor changes in ingredients tend to be acceptable; thus they are considered "nonfixed" formula foods. The companies that produce them generally don't spend much, if any, money on testing (other than the minimum required).

Many of these alternative food companies are "private label," which means they don't manufacture their own food. Simply stated, these "manufactured for" companies have another firm make the food for them, using either the firm's formulas or their own. The quality of the final food obviously depends upon the formula, the manufacturer's quality control, the quality of ingredients, and technical support.

There are some fine nonprofessional alternative foods available. You just need to do a little more investigation to determine how good or bad these companies really are. Even if you have decided that supermarket food is the way to go, knowing that dog food labels don't tell it all, this next step is critical in your dog food evaluation.

RESEARCH

If you want to go all the way, you can call the manufacturer directly and ask questions to help you determine the best possible food for your dog. A list of questions, as well as a list of manufacturers' phone numbers, is on pages 151–153.

Whether you call the manufacturer or not, you should perform the following simple home tests to check out Fido's food.

Home-Testing Dry Food

• Fill a glass with water and drop a few pieces of food into it. You don't want to see a lot of chicken feathers or hair.

• Look at the individual nuggets, checking for consistency of size, shape, density, and color. They should be uniform. If some nuggets crush to powder between your fingers while others remain rock-hard or vary in size, the manufacturer's extruding equipment (which makes the nuggets) is poor, and the product is not likely to be any better.

• Beware of dry dog food bags that feel greasy on the outside. If the fat has soaked through, the manufacturer is probably using poor quality bags, leaving the food susceptible to rodent, insect, and bacterial infestation.

• See if the bottom of the bag contains "fines" (tiny crumbled particles or powder). A small amount is to be expected, but a lot may jeopardize your dog's nutrition. Each nugget contains equal amounts of the mixed and balanced nutrients. The more fines there are, the fewer the whole nuggets, which means reduced or imbalanced nutrition and sloppy manufacturing.

• Smell the food. It shouldn't have a peculiar, moldy, or rancid odor.

• Natural dry food has a shelf life of about nine months. Artificially preserved food can last one year or more past the sell-by date. Look at the date when the food was made. Some dates are coded, so ask someone at the store to help decipher it.

Home-Testing Canned Food

• Be sure there are no swellings or raised bumps on the can. Both usually indicate that the vacuum seal has been broken and the product can be harboring disease-causing bacteria.

• Put the contents of the can into a plate. Cut it into thirds horizontally, from top to bottom. Compare the three sections for consistency in color, and equal distribution of fat and other ingredients. You don't want to see a large glob of fat in the middle. In small cans, fat sometimes rises to the top; this is acceptable.

• Examine the food very well, looking for large pieces of blood vessels, tendons, or ligaments. (They often look like large rubber bands.) You shouldn't find any hair, feathers, or foreign material in the food.

If you haven't selected your dog's present food based on nutritional merits, don't despair. Changing from one food to the other is not difficult, providing you do so slowly, adding a small amount of the new food to the old. Now that you know what to look for in a dog food, you will be able to make an educated selection. To make it even easier for you, I have made the following checklist for dry food:

• It must be 100% nutritional by AAFCO feeding trials.

• It should have 18% minimum protein.

• It should have at least 8% fat.

• Carbohydrates are not included in the gross analysis. You need to add up all the percentages and subtract from 100 to determine the percent of carbs in the food.

- The first seven ingredients should have at least one "meat protein." Meat and bone meal don't count

- The fiber should not be less than 1%.

- It should be manufactured "by" rather than "for."

- It should include feeding directions.

- It should not have dyes or chemical preservatives.

CHAPTER TWO

Mealtime Regimes: The Proper Way to Feed Your Dog

Dogs must eat dog food! And they must eat it on a consistent routine. Two of my closest friends learned this lesson the hard way. They bought a Saint Bernard puppy and promptly named him Big Boy, knowing that once he reached adulthood, he would live up to his name. They decided to "free-feed" (see below) so that he could monitor his own food requirements. Because Big Boy, like most puppies, was more interested in life around him than in his food, he ate only when he was hungry. Fearful that he wasn't getting enough food and wanting him to eat at the same time they did, my friends started to add some of their dinner to his dish. It didn't take long for Big Boy to figure out that some of the food in his dish originated from the dinner table, and that it tasted far better than the dog food he was getting. He soon figured out that all he had to do was sit by the table, put his little paw on their laps, and bat those big brown eyes.

Big Boy ate with them for two years, a practice that came to a sudden and disastrous end during Thanksgiving dinner. My friends tried to get Big Boy to leave the room, but he refused, pulling the tablecloth and all of the dinner—turkey, stuffing, cranberry sauce, gravy, the works—onto the floor. Thanksgiving was ruined for everyone except, of course, Big Boy. My friends had made several mistakes. One was to feed their dog only human food. Another was to let him sit near the dinner table during their mealtimes. Proper mealtime routines are as much about behavior modification for your dog as they are about nutrition.

Whether you have a puppy, adolescent, or senior dog, its mealtime requirements will be similar. While each stage of a dog's life will require some lifestyle adjustments, the basic guidelines for feeding canines remain the same, no matter their shape, color, or size. Although mealtime habits begin to develop the day he's born, once Fido comes to live with you, a new regimen should be established and become the foundation for the rest of his life. You need to make decisions about mealtimes now. Believe it or not, established feeding habits are not going to change much once your puppy becomes an adult, or even as he evolves into a senior. You must remember that you are in charge, no matter how cute, how sweet, or how demanding your dog becomes. Once you determine what to feed, when to feed, how to feed (either with "portion-control" or "free-feed"), you need to be consistent and stick to the routine. Consistency is the key when it comes to mealtimes. Snacks and treats can vary, as long as they have healthy ingredients and are not given as a reward for begging. Begging is not an inherited behavior; it's learned from owners who need to set boundaries by repetition and accept nothing less than good manners.

PORTION-CONTROL VERSUS FREE-FEED VERSUS MEALTIME SERVING

These are the three ways to feed a dog, and since free-feed is closest to the natural feeding of wild dogs and their relatives, that's the one I prefer. In the wild, a pack of dogs chase down their prey, eat what they immediately need after the chase, and return to their rest place with various parts to nibble on until it's time to chase down another meal. When you pour dry food into a bowl and leave it for your dog all day, that method is called free-feed. The quantity poured into the bowl will determine if it is portion-controlled or not.

The only healthy way to free-feed is to portion out the amount of food you are going to leave down all day; thus the term "portion-control free-feed." After reading the label on the bag, use the guidelines on page 29, and pour in the recommended amount of food or what you consider to be required for your puppy or dog throughout the day. You must measure it, so that you know if your dog is eating, how much he is eating, and if the amount has to be adjusted for weight gain or loss. Remember that dogs are like us—their appetite and weight can go up and down, especially puppies. If you pour the entire recommended quantity into the bowl in the morning, you cannot refill until the next morning. If puppies are started out with portion-control free-feeding, they will generally nibble all day, finishing the food when it's just about time for a refill. If you are changing a dog from mealtime servings to portion-control, you will need to divide the entire day into two feedings, morning and night, because that dog will probably eat the entire portioned amount at one time. Within a few weeks the dog should temper himself and nibble throughout the day. If he doesn't adjust, free-feed is not for him or you.

Mealtime serving works best for the finicky dog (if the food isn't eaten within a specified amount of time, it is picked up, refrigerated, and served at the next meal), the gluttonous dog that doesn't control his eating, and the sick or senior dog who requires frequent meals because of the addition of medication or the need to feed a small amount frequently. Just like free-feeding, the amount of food you pour into the bowl for each meal must be measured.

HOW MUCH TO FEED

Caloric requirements vary from dog to dog, even among the same breed. The number of calories a dog requires depends on many factors, including size, age, activity level, and housing conditions. A canine athlete or growing puppy will require more calories than an adult dog of the same breed left at home all day. A senior debilitated dog may require additional calories to avoid weight loss, while another senior may need intense calorie restriction because of his slow metabolism. Smaller dogs generally require more calories per day than larger ones do.

Once you've determined the approximate number of calories your dog needs, divide that into the total amount of calories in his food. Feed that amount for 2 or 3 weeks, after which you need to do the "feel test" (p. 62). If your dog feels overweight, you need to decrease the amount of food you are feeding, and if his ribs are prominent, you need to increase the food intake. As a general rule of thumb, however, the following guidelines apply.

- Small breeds under 5 lbs.: 50 calories per pound per day
- Medium breeds up to 50 lbs.: 40 calories per pound per day
- Large and giant breeds over 50 lbs.: 30 calories per pound per day
- A puppy requires double the calories of an adult
- A pregnant dog requires 1½ to 3 times the calories of an adult.

Example: Mimi is a 5-pound toy poodle. The canned food she is being fed contains 500 calories per 15 oz. can. To determine how much of the can she should be fed daily, multiply Mimi's weight × 50 = 250 calories daily. Since the canned food contains 500 calories, Mimi requires approximately ½ can of food daily, or ¼ can in the morning and ¼ can in the evening.

How to Determine the Calories in Your Dog's Food

If you are cooking for your dog, or your food package doesn't have the recommended feeding requirements, you can calculate the number of calories in his food if you know how many calories the major nutrients contain and the percentage of those nutrients in the food. The number of calories per nutrient breaks down as follows:

1 gram protein = 4 calories

1 gram carbohydrate = 4 calories

1 gram fat = 9 calories

The formula is as follows:

Nutrient percentage × calories per nutrient = calories

For example, take a dog food that has 30% protein, 40% carbs, and 20% fat.

Protein calories = 30 × 4 = 120 calories

Carb calories = 40 × 4 = 160 calories

Fat calories = 20 × 9 = 180 calories

Add them all up, and you have a total of 460 calories per serving.

Feeding Do's

These general tips should help get you started with proper feeding habits.

• Feed a puppy under 4–6 months of age at least 3 times daily or leave a specific amount of dry food available throughout the day.

• Get into the habit of cleaning the water bowl daily, and refilling it as needed.

• Feed a dog over 4–6 months of age 2 times daily or leave a specific amount of dry food throughout the day. Three and 4 daily feedings are reserved for seniors.

• Feedings should be at set times, preferably prior to your own meal. If your dog rejects its meal after a specific amount of time, pick up the dish and save the food for the next meal. If you try to enhance the flavor of the meal, you may be successful the first few times but trust me, eventually *nothing* will taste good enough. Dogs eat to satisfy their needs, sometimes needing more or less food. If your puppy or dog skips a meal or two that's okay, as long as he doesn't appear to be sick.

• Once you've selected the food you are going to feed, stay with that food unless there is a problem with it. If you absolutely must give your dog a home-cooked meal, do so once or twice weekly.

• Large and medium dogs should be fed primarily dry food. While some owners will add water to increase the taste, if you are going to let your dog self-regulate its food during the day, added water can cause the food to go bad.

• When feeding more than one dog, keep them far enough apart to decrease competitive eating. Each dog should have his own food dish. Water can be shared.

• Do give healthy treats. Vegetables cooked or raw, nonbuttered popcorn, vitamin treats, natural biscuits without dyes or preservatives (providing your dog doesn't have to watch his calories), and homemade treats are acceptable.

• When you give a treat make sure that you are the same height as your dog is, or higher. You need to fortify your alpha position.

• If your puppy is teething, put some baby teething rings in the freezer. A frozen teething ring or ice cubes can give puppies some relief.

FEEDING DON'TS

Dogs have been domesticated for over 10,000 years, so you'd think we'd know how to feed them, but many of us still haven't learned. What follows are definite no-no's when it comes to feeding your dog or puppy.

1. Once-a-day feeding is wrong for dogs, big or small. Digestion starts in the mouth and finishes in the intestines. A very hungry dog will not chew its food, thus bypassing the first stage of digestion, which includes breaking the food down mechanically through chewing and with the enzymes the saliva. An older dog produces less enzymes, probably can't chew well, and will therefore need supplemental help. While chewing a dry food doesn't guarantee cleaner teeth, there are some foods that are formulated to clean as the dog chews. A hungry dog gulps and swallows. A fast-eating dog ingests air as well as food. Besides indigestion, swallowed air can create *bloat*, a potentially deadly condition in deep-chested and large dogs.

2. Feeding a diet of *only* canned food may not be fair to you or your dog. Canned food can consist of 75–78% water, leaving very little room in the can for the actual building blocks of nutrition. Depending on the brand of canned food, a 40-pound dog can require as many as 4 cans of food daily to get the proper level of nutrition, which I'm willing to bet you are not feeding. If you are not feeding the required amount, chances are your dog is not be as healthy he should be. Canned food generally contains more fat than dry food. Dogs with digestive problems can have loose stools or diarrhea. Canned food, as a rule, certainly tastes better than dry. If your dog inhales his food, canned food is simply not for him. Canned food should not be left out all day. If you are free-feeding, you can't use canned. It can attract insects or spoil.

3. Don't allow table scraps or homemade diets you've simply thrown together (especially all-meat) to replace a store-bought dog food. Not only are you jeopardizing your dog's health, you're spoiling him. If you add more than 25% table scraps to a well-balanced food, there's a real chance of upsetting that balance.

4. Unless your dog has the metabolism of the Tasmanian devil, you can't just pour an arbitrary amount of food into a dish. Besides overfeeding and making your pet fat, if you don't know how much food was in the dish when you filled it, how will you know if your dog is eating or not? Sometimes the only way we can tell a dog is not feeling well is by the quantity of food he's eating. Free-feed portion-control the recommended quantity and adjust by adding or subtracting, depending on your dog's weight.

5. Feeding raw meat can be dangerous to your dog's health. It can contain bacteria, their harmful toxins, and parasites. If you want some names of the health villains that are generally destroyed through cooking, they include *E. coli*, Camptobacteria, Salmonella, and trichinosis. Dogs and their relatives can eat raw meat in the wild because it is freshly killed and has not been contaminated at the slaughterhouse, shipping dock, and store. If you absolutely must feed a raw meat diet, it must be frozen so that some of the villains are destroyed, it must be balanced by a nutritionist, and the company must supply you with evidence that it tests for the mentioned bacteria.

6. Adding supplements indiscriminately to your dog's food can unbalance the formulation of the food. Check chapter 3, and the appendixes on vitamins, minerals, and herbs at the back of the book, before you begin adding supplements.

7. If you change brands of food, do so slowly and gradually to tolerance. A sudden change can cause gastrointestinal problems such as loose stools or diarrhea, gas, vomiting or constipation.

8. Never reduce your dog's quantity of food below 25% of the amount recommended by the manufacturer or by your calculations. The recommended amount of food to be fed has been calculated by the manufacturer, based on its food formulation, to deliver the minimum daily requirements for the average dog. While your dog may not be average, if you reduce the amount of food beyond ¼ the recommended amount, you are jeopardizing your dog's nutrition. If you are cutting back on the food because of weight gain, then you will have to change foods, perhaps to a "light" form. If you are cutting back because you simply can't believe that your dog requires all the bag states, then change to a better-quality food that will require less quantity.

FEEDING PREGNANT OR LACTATING MOMS

Dogs can be bred after their first heat (although I prefer their second) all the way through their early middle years. Once your female has veterinarian approval for mating, it's time to consider feeding her and treating her like a mom, even before the actual conception. Since she carries the puppies for only two months, it's easy to understand that her body requires all the nutritional building blocks beforehand. She should be fed a high-quality alternative professional food (see p. 23). Any type of nutritional inadequacy or imbalance can ruin a healthy litter. Proper supplementation is a must to ensure the addition of nutrients that may not be available in the dog food. Chapter 3 tells you all you need to know about supplementing, as do the appendixes on vitamins, minerals, and herbs at the back of this book.

During the First Month

Mom can be fed with either the free-feeding or portion-control methods. Just don't let her gain too much weight. During her first month, her ribs should be easily detectable, with just a pinch of fat and muscle covering them. Quantities of food will probably change from week to week, depending on exercise, number of snacks, number of puppies, etc. Since thirst will vary, fresh and clean water is essential. If you are adding red raspberry to her water, clean the bowl and refill it daily.

If Mom is not in the habit of exercising, this is the time to start, increasing the length of exercise time as her body becomes more conditioned. Swimming, hide-and-seek, fetch, and long walks are all healthy exercises. Rewards should consist of nonfattening treats: carrots, apples, and celery. Even though raisins and cheese are high in calories, their iron and calcium content makes them Mom's treat of choice.

The Second and Last Month

This is when your dog will finally start to look like a mom. Like any pregnant female, her waistline will soon disappear, she will become increasingly hungry, and chances are you will see personality changes as well. Whatever brand of food you are feeding, you need to change to the puppy form. Since puppy food is more concentrated than adult, she may be less uncomfortable with smaller amounts of food in her stomach. If you are feeding her with the mealtime method, it's time to add an additional meal or two, increasing her food little by little so that the nutritional needs of her and the puppies are satisfied without making Mom fat. If you're free-feeding portion-controlled, increase her total quantity daily, being careful not to make her fat. Since change can promote gastrointestinal disturbances, don't change food brands or make other radical changes at this point.

Because her appetite will increase day by day (until close to delivery), but her desire to exercise will decrease, treats need to be healthy but non-fattening. Good choices include fresh vegetables, freeze-dried beef or chicken treats, low-fat cheese, and—believe it or not—the high-quality protein and low fat of dried fish treats (for cats). Salty treats are out.

When at last her hunger subsides, and she rejects her meals, it's probably delivery time. Don't force her to eat, make sure she has fresh water and your moral support. She and her puppies will be fine. As her appetite returns to normal 1–2 days after delivery, keep feeding her just as you have been, paying close attention to her ribs and waistline, and adjusting her amount of puppy food accordingly. As the puppies grow and demand more milk, she will require more food.

During Lactation

Whether there is 1 puppy or 12, lactation can be trying. Sometimes moms will stop eating; they just don't seem to have an appetite. This is the dangerous time when owners spoil their dogs by adding one food after the other to entice them to eat. If your veterinarian has declared Mom and puppies healthy, she will eat when she is hungry.

Don't worry about her calcium level either. All major-brand puppy foods contain more than enough for Mom and the puppies. If you absolutely must do something about it, offer her lactose-free milk, cottage cheese, yogurt, and eggs as daily snacks between meals. Whatever you do, don't let her con you into feeding them in place of balanced food.

FEEDING PUPPIES WITHOUT A MOM

A substitute lactating dog, even though she is a stranger, is optimum. It is essential that the puppy gets the first milk (colostrum) within 24–48 hours of birth, which the substitute may be able to provide. If that is not possible, then you will have to become the mom. Colostrum is now being sold through veterinarians and health food stores, so you can add it to the formula for the first week.

You'll have to serve frequent meals, as often as every two hours being optimum. Keep the puppies warm by placing them on a heating pad (with no access to the wire) set on low, and run a vaporizer in the room. Since there is no canine mom, you have to weigh each puppy on a gram scale to make sure it is gaining weight, feed it by bottle or eyedropper, and then place it back in its den after cleaning its mouth and other end with a damp cloth or tissue. The easiest part of playing mom is buying the milk substitute or making it. I recommend buying one of the brands available in your pet store or through your veterinarian. Those formulas have the additional nutrients your homemade formula will lack. Remember, the formula you are feeding should resemble mom's milk, so heat the portion you will be feeding to room temperature. Check the temperature by putting some of the formula on your wrist. If it's okay there, it's fine to feed it to the puppies. Just like with human babies.

If you don't have experience hand-feeding puppies, ask your veterinarian to show you. All you will have to do is hold the puppy as you would a baby (supporting its head), and allow it to suck from the bottle. If it isn't sucking, then small amounts of liquid need to be squeezed from an eyedropper that is placed in the side of the puppy's mouth—*being very careful to make sure it doesn't enter the windpipe*. Slow and easy is the best approach. While it's impossible for me to tell you how much to feed the puppy, 10–20 milliliters per feeding is a good place to start. It's better to underfeed than to give too much. Once you've done it a few times, you will be able to judge if the puppy is full by the increased size of the abdomen, and eventually gauge the amount of formula by that. Don't handle the puppy after it has eaten, except to wipe its behind with a damp cloth to stimulate defecation. Place it gently back on the heating pad. If you want to make a homemade formula, see page 149 under *Recipes*.

WEANING PUPPIES

Early weaning is selfish and unnatural, unless the health of the mother is at stake. Puppies require the easy-to-digest, nutrient-packed milk from their mother or formula until 6 weeks of age. Early weaning can create all types of health problems, including food allergies, during their adult life. If you keep Mom's puppy food (canned or dry) in a shallow dish, the inquisitive puppies are sure to walk into the food, smell it, and eventually try to eat it! They will also start to lap water as they fall in it and play around it. To prevent drowning, it's essential to put the water in a shallow spillproof dish, then clean and refill it as often as needed.

If Feeding Mom Dry Puppy Food

Fill another shallow dish with puppy food and add enough water to soften it (making it the consistency of oatmeal). Just as with Mom's hard food, the puppies will eventually end up in the dish, lapping the "mush" that tastes just like Mom's milk. Timing is everything. At this stage Mom is tired, sore, and in need of escape. Once the puppies start to eat on their own, they will demand less milk from Mom, and give her the chance to leave the den for longer intervals. Day by day you will decrease the additional water until the puppies are eating solid puppy food, free-feed. That's when Mom and the puppies can celebrate their independence.

If Feeding Mom Canned Puppy Food

Simply add water until the food becomes a mush. Day by day you will decrease additional water until you are serving direct from the can (heated to room temperature). Since canned food can spoil, you will need to refill the bowls frequently.

With No Mom

Once the puppies reach 4–6 weeks or have become brave enough to investigate beyond their den, it's time to add a puppy food (dry or canned) to the formula. Start with ¼ puppy food and ¾ formula. Don't add too much additional water because you will dilute the puppy's meal. Day by day you add more puppy food and less formula until you are feeding only puppy food. Congratulations, job well done, Mom!

FEEDING THE YOUNG AND MIDDLE-AGED DOG

As your puppy grows into early years, adolescence, and young adulthood, you will have to modify some of your feeding habits, but within the realm of my basic feeding rules. Be prepared for the young puppy and adult to reject its meals because life is simply too exciting. Biscuits and treats must be stopped so that your young dog doesn't insist on making them the most important part of his life. Rewards in training sessions can be vitamin treat supplements, since these (p. 155) are a must for the poor eater anyway. While your dog's poor appetite may concern you, it's actually a healthy preventive against fast growth and the corresponding bone problems fat, fast-growing young dogs can develop. Your dog will fill out and look his part when he matures at age 2 or 3. As he

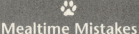

Mealtime Mistakes

Dairy Products May Not Be Right for Your Dog. While it's true that milk and cheese are excellent sources of protein and fat, they can cause diarrhea in an adult dog. Dogs can develop lactose intolerance just as we can.

Too Much Liver Can Be Harmful. While liver contains myriad nutritional components, a daily diet of liver can cause diarrhea or vitamin A and D toxicity.

Don't Turn Your Dog into a Vegetarian. Your dog evolved as a meat eater and needs to continue to be. For his wolf relatives, small and medium animals form their diet of choice. While grass is included in their diet, dogs and wolves evolved with canine teeth to tear flesh and enzymes to break down meats. Even though it is available in stores, an all-vegetarian diet will not make dogs healthier.

Fat Scraps Are Not Healthy. While it may help the coat shine, fat can make your dog fat, and cause pancreatic disease and diarrhea. Your dog should receive plenty of fat from his dog food. If his coat needs help, see pages 8, 11, 112, 115, 157, 158.

Never Leave Your Dog Without Water. Never restrict your dog's water intake. If urination within the house is a problem, then it's time to confine your pet to a crate or a room that's easy to clean, lined with newspapers. Dogs dehydrate easily, and need plenty of water.

Mealtime Mistakes

Don't Feed Dogs from Plastic Dishes. While they may not break easily, plastic dishes can cause a sensitivity or allergic reaction on your dog's chin, harbor bacteria, and retain odors that can cause a finicky dog to reject his meal. Metal or ceramic dishes are your best choice.

Don't Feed Your Dog from Combined Food and Water Dishes. Unless your dog has the table manners of Emily Post, some of the food is bound to end up in the water, creating a haven for bacteria growth.

Bloat-Prone Dogs Should Not Be Eating from a Dish on the Floor. Elevate the dish on a table or stand so that the food is at shoulder level. Your dog will swallow less air and have a more pleasant dining experience. See box on p. 73.

Don't Teach Your Dog to Beg. As mentioned before, dogs are taught to beg, either intentionally or otherwise. Feeding scraps occasionally will only teach them to want more. The more often you succumb to his pleas, the more your dog will beg.

Don't Mix and Match Quality. In other words, don't add a high-quality canned food to a dry food that's not manufactured by the same company.

Don't Oversupplement. Don't get carried away with adding one supplement after another. Read chapter 3 to find out how much, and check the appendixes

grows in height, his feeding dish must be raised to keep it at shoulder height to prevent bloat.

FEEDING THE SENIOR DOG

Except for the fact that a senior dog may be set in his ways, and unhealthy ones at that, seniors need to follow the same rules the younger ones do; with some exceptions:

• Frequent smaller meals will aid digestion.

• The higher-quality the protein, the better; and it shouldn't be reduced unless a veterinarian tells you to.

• If a significant number of teeth have been lost, canned food should be fed.

• Vegetable enzymes will aid digestion.

• Since some seniors lose their sense of smell, you may want to add a strong-smelling canned food to the regular food, dry or canned. If your vet's biannual exam hasn't uncovered kidney disease, the addition of an inexpensive fish or chicken cat food can turn a humdrum meal into a gourmet delight. It's an excellent way to sneak in the various supplements or medications your senior will need.

• Some senior dogs have a tendency to gain weight. Their food should include moderate to low quantities of fat.

• If you can't seem to reduce your senior to his once svelte shape and weight, reevaluate his food requirements according to the manufacturer or by calculating the number of calories he needs to look good again. Set a goal. Then follow my diet plan for weight loss, pages 62–71, until you have reached your goal.

• Watch his water intake carefully. Diabetes and kidney disease, common in seniors, cause tremendous thirst.

• Treats must be low-salt, preferably vitamin supplements or raw vegetables.

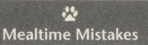

Mealtime Mistakes

at the back of this book for more detailed recommendations.

Don't Exercise Right Away. Wait at least one hour after eating before taking your dog for his nightly or morning walk or run. It doesn't matter if your dog is big or small.

CHAPTER THREE

Supplements for Healthier Dogs

Breeding the perfect dog takes diligence, money, and time, sometimes generations. Once a breeder has succeeded in producing the type of dog he wants, it's off to the Westminster Kennel Club show and beyond. But sometimes, in the quest for the "perfect" specimen, breeders can get carried away. "Gail," a husky breeder, perfected the rich black-and-white coat. "David," a Rottweiler breeder, bred generations of Rotts with perfect chests and mild personalities. A golden retriever breeder was able to develop "bone-disease-free" litters, even though goldens are notorious for bone disease. And finally, a chihuahua breeder had bred perfect little show winners with beautiful healthy skin. All of this was accomplished with available dog food, but all of these breeders thought that they could do a bit better with supplements.

Both Gail and David thought additional calcium was required, so Gail added bone meal to her husky's high-quality alternative food, and David added "just a little" calcium powder to the same brand of dog food. The additional calcium caused such body chaos that the dogs' coats turned bright, vibrant red! The golden breeder experimented with several multivitamin–mineral supplements until she realized that the probable cause of her dogs' newly acquired cases of bone disease was these supplements. Finally, the innocent chihuahua breeder who fed a high-quality food, then added a "good" helping of skin and coat supplement, succeeded in producing the fattest little hairy dogs you'd ever want to see. If only they had left well enough alone, or read this chapter first!

This chapter is intended as a guide for supplementing the diet of a dog that is basically healthy, or whose condition would benefit from a supplemental nutritional program, such as a pregnant or lactating mom. If your dog has a either a specific or a general health problem, turn to chapter 4 for nutritional advice on a range of general ill-health conditions.

All of the supplements recommended in this chapter are covered in detail in Appendix A, "Vitamins and Minerals," and Appendix B, "Herbs, Grasses, and Other Natural Supplements." Once you spot what you need, read up on the individual supplement for more detailed information.

SUPPLEMENTING SUPERMARKET FOODS

Although supermarket foods are formulated well and deliver the basic nutritional requirements for the average dog, most dogs are not average, and the canine nutritional requirements presented by the pet food industry simply do not include all the nutrients needed for all breeds. The addition of a synthetic supplement is less likely to affect the overall formulation of a supermarket food than of an alternative professional food. Supermarket foods generally give the owner a margin of "supplementation error" so that the additional nutrients don't ruin the balance of the food. Since increasing the nutritive value of these foods is a must for optimum health, if you're not adding a grass or natural whole food, then you should be supplementing with a wide-spectrum vitamin–mineral supplement and a digestive enzyme.

SUPPLEMENTING ALTERNATIVE FOODS

Professional alternative foods need to be supplemented more conservatively. Although these foods tend to concentrate more nutrients in the individual nuggets or the can, they still need to be supplemented. It can be unwise, however, to add a synthetic vitamin or mineral supplement to them because the delicate balance of that expensive, well-balanced food can be upset. The additional nutrients can confuse the digestive process. The best way to supplement these foods is to add natural whole foods (grass, algae, bee pollen, etc.).

If you look at the food your dog would be eating were it in the wild or living 10,000 years ago, his diet would include the partially digested grass and various plants eaten by rabbits or small herbivores the dog eats. Although vitamin C is made in the liver of dogs, additional C, antioxidants, enzymes, and other nutrients are important to a dog's health. Antioxidants, which occur in high amounts in plants, are not new; they are simply newly discovered.

VITAMINS

Vitamins are organic substances, found in minute quantities in foods, that are essential to normal life functioning in all animals. With few exceptions they cannot be manufactured in the body and must be obtained through diet or supplements. Some vitamins, including A, beta-carotene, C, and E, are known as antioxidants. These protect the body from potentially injurious by-products that form in the body every day, causing all types of diseases. As mentioned, the vitamins and minerals that dogs require, their benefits, dosages, etc., are listed in Appendix A. Vitamins can be found at your local pet supply store or at your vet, in pill, liquid, or paste form.

HERBS AND OTHER NATURAL SUPPLEMENTS

Herbs, grasses, and other natural foods (e.g., bee pollen, seaweed) have marvelous curative properties. Because of its complex array of nutritional components, an herbal remedy is selected for a specific problem and, at the same time, to support the rest of the body or portions of it, so that healing can occur. Natural medicine approaches disease as an imbalance in the body. It maintains that a "healthy" body should not become diseased, so that treating just the ill portion of the body, as we do with modern medicines, is incorrect. Herbalists believe that the body can heal the imbalance itself if given the right tools (nutrients).

Whether you're a first-time dog owner or a veteran breeder, there are many problems that benefit from the holistic or total natural approach to healing. The puppy with ringworm or mange, or the senior dog with arthritis, is a candidate for the natural medicine approach. While one can cure ringworm and mange with drugs, or give relief from arthritis with aspirin and other painkillers, the herbal options also work, but in a different way. The appropriate herbs will build up the immune system of the puppy so it can fight off the skin disease, and will support the stiff sore joints so that the degeneration slows down and the toxic wastes within the joints are eliminated. Remedies for specific health problems are covered in chapter 4. If you're looking for a veterinarian who specializes in holistic healing, you can call the Association of Holistic Veterinarians at (410) 569-0795.

If you're looking for a general, daily supplement, I always prefer the "natural form" rather than a formula made in a laboratory. Nature knows best, especially when it comes to balancing those micronutrients we know so little about. Since most supplements are added to your dog's already balanced dog food, you must be careful not to upset that carefully developed ratio of vitamins, minerals, and all the other nutrients that are in your dog's bowl. There is less chance of upsetting the balance when supplementing with a natural food rather than a synthetic combination of nutrients.

Supplement Rules

1. When adding a new supplement to your dog's mealtime routine, introduce one at a time. Wait 3–5 days to see if there are any side effects, such as differences in bowel movements or changes in skin/hair.

2. Never add a multivitamin–mineral supplement to an alternative high-quality food unless the supplement is a "natural whole food." See Appendix B, page 136.

3. Never mix one "whole natural food" with another. Schedule one in any dog food at one meal and the other in another meal.

3. Whatever type of supplement you use, your dog's opinion counts. If he won't eat it, don't force him to eat it. The dog's failure to accept the supplement is the no. 1 cause of poor results. Look for treats, wafers, biscuits, tasty tablets; your dog will love all of them. Powders or liquids might be acceptable to your dog. You may want to hide the supplement in peanut butter, cream cheese, etc.

4. Never give more than the recommended amount unless otherwise directed.

5. Don't give more than one supplement at a time unless you are certain they belong together.

6. Make sure the supplement is fresh and is stored as recommended.

Recommended Supplemental Programs

For general, day-to-day improved health, I've developed the following supplemental programs. These are designed for overall well-being, not to correct a specific illness or problem. The latter is treated in chapter 4. For most of these, I list the recommended supplements, then how to supply each one. For dosages, I've generalized dogs into small, medium, and large breeds. These are defined as follows:

Small breed: ranges from the very small (2 lbs.) to 20–25 lbs.

Medium breed: ranges from 25 to 50 lbs.

Large/giant breed: ranges from 50 to 100 lbs.

I included giant with the large breed because, for the purposes of this book, their nutritional management is similar to that of large breeds.

Puppies over 6 Weeks

Puppies need a well-balanced vitamin–mineral supplement to ensure adequate nutrient intake and a vegetable digestive enzyme to ensure nutrient absorption and utilization.

How to Supply It: These can be supplied with a general multivitamin–mineral supplement that comes in the form of a treat, paste, or wafer. It should be given between meals unless otherwise directed. Or you can use a vitamin–mineral supplement coupled with (or without amino) acids and fatty acids in powder or liquid form. Add it directly to supermarket food. Do not add to an alternative high-quality food. Instead, provide an extra meal of cottage cheese, yogurt, chopped meat, etc., plus the supplement. Follow directions for dosage.

The third option is to add a natural "whole food" to any puppy food: bee pollen, brewer's yeast, spirulina, algae, wheat or oat or barley grass. Small breeds get ⅛ teaspoon or per directions; medium breeds, ¼ teaspoon or per directions; large breeds, ½ tsp. or per directions. As for the vegetable digestive enzymes, use Prozyme or Florazyme in every meal to increase the amount of nutrition your pet gets from its food.

Young, Healthy Adults

The age range for this category is based on the size of the breed. For small breeds, a young adult is from 6 months to 8 years; the range is from 1 to 6 years for medium and large breeds. Young adult dogs are in their prime, and require a well-balanced vitamin–mineral supplement to ensure adequate nutrition. An antioxidant is also recommended, as is a vegetable digestive enzyme to increase the amount of nutrition your pet gets from its food.

How To Supply It: A general vitamin–mineral supplement should be available in treat, paste, or wafer form, and given between meals. Or you can use a vitamin–mineral supplement coupled with (or without) amino acids and fatty acids in a powder or liquid form. Add it directly to supermarket food. Do not add it directly to an alternative quality food. Instead, provide an extra meal of table scraps, cottage cheese, yogurt, etc., plus the supplement. Follow dosage directions. Another option is a natural "whole food," rich in antioxidants, added to any dog food. Spirulina, algae, alfalfa, and oat or wheat or barley grass are excellent antioxidant supplements. Dosage for small breeds is ¼ tsp. or per directions; for medium breeds, ½ tsp. or per directions; for large breeds, ¾–1 tsp. or per directions

Another suggestion for antioxidants is to find a commercial formulation including several antioxidants and their support nutrients that can be added to supermarket food. Do not add it directly to an alternative quality food. If it's in a treat, paste, or wafer form, give it between meals. If it's in powder or liquid form, add it to an extra meal of cottage cheese, yogurt, etc. Follow dosage directions.

Finally, Prozyme or Florazyme can be added in every meal, as directed, to aid digestion.

Pregnant or Lactating Dogs

Pregnant or lactating dogs can benefit from red raspberry infusion or tea, which should be started at the 40th–50th day. Kelp, other seaweed, or dandelion (fresh or tincture) should be given as an additional natural source of calcium. Don't combine raspberry and kelp with a natural "whole food" or multivitamin–mineral supplement. They can be combined with vegetable enzymes. Give the pregnancy/lactating supplements in one meal, and the other supplements in another.

How To Supply It: Red raspberry infusion or tea for six weeks after the 40th day. Small breeds, 1 tsp. twice daily in food; medium breeds, 1½–2 tsp. twice daily in food; large breeds, 3 tsp. twice daily in food.

Kelp can be given in liquid form. Dosage for small breeds, one drop daily in food or water; for medium breeds, 2 drops daily in food or water; for large breeds, 2–3 drops daily in food or water.

Dandelion is available in health food stores. If you're using cut or crushed fresh leaves, the dosage for small dogs is ⅛ tsp. in food; for medium dogs, ¼ tsp.; for large dogs, ½–1 tsp. Tinctures vary in potency, so check the directions, which are generally given in adult dog dosages. Because these are young adults, err on the safe side. For small dogs, use ⅛–¼ the recommended adult dosage; for medium dogs, use ½ the recommended adult dosage; and for large dogs, you can administer the full adult dosage.

Geriatric Dogs

The term "geriatric" generally refers to the age at which a dog's body starts to show the effects of aging; a degenerative process that begin years before any physical changes actually show. A majority of small and medium breeds will start to show signs of aging at the age of 8: arthritis, cataract formation, gray hairs, slower metabolism, etc. Large breeds start to show signs of aging much earlier, at 5–6 years: gray muzzles, early heart disease, arthritis, etc. One of the goals of this book is to slow down the degenerative changes, keeping your dog healthier and happier long into his senior years.

Geriatric or senior dogs need a general multivitamin–mineral supplement that contains amino acids to ensure adequate protein. They also need omega-3 fatty acids for a healthy immune system, and to help combat aches and pains; potassium-rich herbs (pages 138, 143) or "complete foods"; a vegetable digestive enzyme; an antioxidant supplement to slow down the aging process, help sore joints, and prevent disease; and a bone protection nutrient (p. 52) for arthritis and hip dysplasia. Large breeds need all of the above plus "whole foods" or herbs rich in taurine and L-carnitine.

How to Supply It: A general vitamin–mineral supplement with amino acids in a wafer, paste, or treat form can be given between meals. Or use a vitamin–mineral supplement with amino acids and fatty acids (omega-3 is preferable) in powder or liquid form. Add it to the supermarket food. Do not add it directly to an alternative high-quality food. If it's in powder or liquid form, add it to an extra meal containing cottage cheese, yogurt, etc.

As another option, use a "natural complete food" that is particularly rich in potassium and protein: brewer's yeast and garlic, torula yeast and garlic, spirulina, or bee pollen. Dosages for these whole foods are small dogs, ⅛–¼ tsp. in food daily; medium dogs, ½ tsp. in food daily; large dogs, 1 tbsp. in food daily.

Omega-3 fatty acids can be found in oil of primrose, flaxseed oil, and fish oil, all of which must be given in conjunction with an antioxidant. I prefer the omega-3 supplements that are already combined with the proper antioxidants. These include NutriVed O.F.A. chewable tablets (veterinarian only), Derm Caps (veterinarian only), OptiCoat 11, and my own Essential Gold chewable tablets. If you are adding just the omega-3 oils, you must include a "whole food supplement" rich in antioxidants (spirulina, alfalfa) or an antioxidant or antioxidant combination. Dosage for small dogs, 150–200 mg. daily; medium dogs, 250–500 mg. daily; large dogs, not to exceed 1,000 mg. daily.

Chopped raw garlic found in the produce section is also recommended as a supplement. Dosages are small dogs, ⅛ tsp. of raw garlic or ¼ small clove in food; medium breed dogs, ¼–½ tsp. raw garlic or ½–1 clove garlic in food; large dogs, ¾–1 tsp. raw garlic or 2 cloves of garlic in food.

Dandelion is recommended to keep the liver and kidney healthy in the older dog and to help shed or prevent those extra pounds that tend to add up as a dog gets older. Dosage is the same as for pregnant/lactating dogs (above).

Cider vinegar is another supplement that is perfect for the older dog. It supplies the additional potassium required, and keeps the body's metabolism in balance. Dosage: ½–1 tsp. plus ½ tsp.-1 tsp. warmed honey per pint of water or in food (not in a metal bowl).

Use Prozyme or Florazyme as directed with every meal, as a vegetable digestive enzyme supplement to aid digestion.

You can add a "natural whole food" rich in antioxidants—spirulina, alfalfa, oat or wheat or barley grass—to food. For small dogs, ¼ tsp. per meal; medium dogs, ½ tsp. per meal; large dogs, ¾–1 tsp. per meal. As an alternative, an antioxidant formulation such as Nu-Pet or Cell Advance (vet only) that includes more than one antioxidant and support nutrients can be added directly to supermarket food. Do not add it to alternative high-quality food. Give as a paste, wafer, or treat between meals. If it is in liquid or powder form, add it to an extra meal of cottage cheese, yogurt, etc. Use recommended dosage.

Taurine and L-carnitine are amino acids that protect the heart (older animals have a high incidence of heart disease) and help stabilize the nervous system (they may help decrease senility).

Taurine can be given by an extra meal of clams, cooked liver or kidney, or cooked tuna 3 times weekly. Small dogs need 100–200 mg. weekly; medium dogs, 200–400 mg. weekly; large dogs, 500–1,000 mg. weekly. This translates into 1 small liver steak for small dogs, 2 good-sized liver steaks for medium dogs, and 3–4 good sized liver steaks for large dogs. Also, for small dogs, ⅛ lb. cooked clams (no shells); for medium dogs, ¼–½ lb. cooked clams; for large dogs, ¾–1 lb. cooked clams.

L-carnitine can be found in both muscle meats and organ meats. Small dogs need 100–150 mg. daily. Medium dogs need about 250 mg., and large dogs require 500 mg.

If your dog has Arthritis (pain, stiffness) which is common in older dogs, I recommend that you discuss this supplementation with your family veterinarian. Give chondroitin sulfate, sea mussels, glucosamine sulfate, or cosequin daily. Glucosamine dosage for small dogs is 200 mg. daily; for medium dogs, 500 mg. daily; for large dogs, 1,000 mg. daily. Include an antioxidant "whole food" such as alfalfa. Alfalfa dosage for small dogs is ¼–½ tsp.; for medium dogs, ½–¾ tsp.; for large dogs, 1 tbsp. daily.

Debilitated Dogs

Sick or recovering dogs needs supplements, but only after you consult with your vet. They need energy supplements; electrolytes (sodium, potassium, magnesium, etc.); additional protein and fatty acids; B vitamins; garlic to strengthen the immune system and supply potassium; antioxidants; acidophilus; and vegetable enzymes. Arthritis doesn't have to turn your once lively dog into a couch potato. Chondroitin sulfate, glucosamine sulfate, cosequin, or sea mussels can provide relief from pain and decrease the degeneration of the joints. Sea mussels (my preference) is a "whole food" that contains the other substances, all capable of keeping the bone structure within the joints healthier.

How To Supply It: For energy, warmed honey or blackstrap molasses to taste is a good natural source of energy. You can also get energy pastes from a vet or specialty pet food catalogs. Administer between meals, 2–4 times a day.

For electrolytes, use Pedialyte or Gatorade. These can be added to the drinking water or given separately.

For a general multivitamin–mineral supplement, use a natural "whole food" that includes spirulina or bee pollen. Dosage for small dogs is ⅛–¼ tsp. daily; for medium breeds, ½ tsp. daily; for large breeds, 1 tablespoon daily. Or use a vitamin, mineral, amino acid, and fatty acid supplement for dogs as directed.

For additional B vitamins, use brewer's or torula yeast as a treat or add it to any dog food, or give a multiple B vitamin supplement for dogs. Dosage is the same as above for spirulina and bee pollen.

To add garlic, use crushed raw garlic from your grocery store, or brewer's yeast and garlic tablets.

Antioxidant-rich natural "whole foods" include alfalfa, algae, and oat or wheat or barley grass. Add these to any type of regular dog food. Follow the recommended dosage.

Acidophilus can be found in powder or liquid form (health food stores) and should be added to every meal. Dosage for small dogs is ¼ recommended adult dose; for medium dogs, ½ recommended adult dose; for large dogs, adult dosage.

For vegetable enzymes, use Prozyme or Florazyme. The dosage of Prozyme is ¼ teaspoon per cup of food.

CHAPTER FOUR

Nutritional Aids for Health and Behavior Problems

During my early years as a veterinarian, I began to notice a peculiar trend. Sometimes, when some symptoms or illness no longer responded to drugs, a well-balanced diet with selected supplements worked where the drugs had failed. Diets and supplements also seemed to enhance the effectiveness of some medical treatments. To me, it was simple logic that dictated the necessity of combining medicine with nutrition. After all, every cell, tissue, and organ of an animal's body is totally dependent on the individual nutritional building blocks derived from food. How could anyone expect a dog to fight off a disease, with or without medicines, if its immune system doesn't have the components it needs to do its job?

If you've turned to this chapter, it means that your dog is suffering from a mild illness or condition that may benefit from proper nutrition. Once your vet has determined your dog's actual health status, or if you've administered your own test per the home health checkup (p. 3), you can then take the necessary nutritional steps to bring him back to the high quality of health he deserves. Some of the solutions in this chapter are behavior-related—for example, anxiety or shyness. Just remember that this book is not meant to replace your family veterinarian. You should consult your vet on any illness, and discuss the nutritional aids I describe with your vet to make sure they don't conflict with any medical treatment he or she may have prescribed.

GENERAL HEALTH AND BEHAVIORAL PROBLEMS

As I mentioned, this book is not meant to replace your family veterinarian or behaviorist. However, I've selected the most common medical and behavioral problems that respond quite well to natural remedies. If you don't find the information here, turn to Appendix E, "Problems/Solution Quick Reference Guide," which will tell you where to get help in this book for specific problems. Keep in mind that the diseases and behavioral problems in this chapter may require a face-to-face visit with a specialist; however, you now have an arsenal of alternative treatments to discuss with him or her.

Allergies

A healthy immune system is designed to recognize and eliminate any foreign protein or other substance from the body. When the immune system overreacts (which can cause harm to the animal), that reaction is termed an *allergy* or *sensitivity*. While veterinarians and allergists distinguish between the two terms based on their chemical reactions, the dog and its owner don't. All they know is that the dog is uncomfortable and has problems: excessive biting and scratching, hives, hair loss, vomiting or diarrhea, runny eyes, bronchitis, asthma, sore ears, chin acne, etc. It is obvious that something does not agree with the dog. The foreign agent may have entered the body via the following means:

• Ingestion of food ingredients, herbs, or medications

• Inhalation of airborne substances (pollens, smoke, dust, dust mites, feathers, mold, toxins, etc.)

• Body contact with grass, carpet, soap, lotions, flea-control products, etc.

• Injection of insect venom.

Pinpointing Allergy Type: Determining that a condition is an allergy or sensitivity rather than a real disease takes veterinary know-how. Once your veterinarian is sure that the symptoms are due to a reaction, it's your job to play Sherlock Holmes and discover the substance that is causing your dog to overreact. The easiest way is to limit your dog's exposure to any substance that might cause a reaction. A contact allergy/sensitivity generally creates symptoms *at the point of contact*. Food, injection and airborne substances can create any of the symptoms mentioned above. Contact allergy or sensitivity will generally cause an area to become irritated, itchy, swollen, or otherwise abnormal-looking. Depending on the area involved, keep the dog away from anything that would touch it. If your dog's belly is irritated, chances are he's lying on something that he shouldn't be. Keep him off grass, carpets, bedding, etc. until the reaction calms down. If his chin is red, change food bowls.

Ingestion allergy or sensitivity can cause gastrointestinal or skin problems. The most common allergy-causing food ingredients include milk, cheese, chicken, soy, and beef. Go back to basics, serving your dog a food with a protein he has never eaten before and a gluten-free carbohydrate (rice or potatoes). The home-cooked food elimination diet (p. 149), can be fed for up to two weeks, but no longer, because it doesn't include all the essential nutrients your dog needs. If you need to go longer term, there are several nonallergenic dog foods fortified with vitamins and minerals available, including those from Nature's Recipe called Innovative Diet (duck and potato or venison and potato), available only from your veterinarian. Other veterinarian balanced diets for allergic dogs include Eukanuba Fish & Potato, Hills Lamb & Rice, and the new Purina CNM dermatology-management diets. All of these products are balanced for long-term use and don't have any potential allergy causing ingredients (brewer's yeast, gluten, corn, etc.) that most foods contain. Investigating the cause of allergy requires that you feed only the one food you have selected *and nothing more.* That means no rawhide, treats of any types, people food, etc. If your dog is used to treats, put some of the nonallergenic dry food in a treat container and make believe. Only monthly heartworm pills, other medications, and fresh water are allowed. If your dog's symptoms are the result of something in the food(s) you were feeding, positive results should be seen in from one week to one month.

Inhalant or injection allergies are the most difficult to determine. Blood tests are available, but they are costly and can be inaccurate. Skin testing is your best bet, but it is expensive and time-consuming. The following is an allergy protocol to help rebalance your dog's immune system. Start with the first, adding the others depending on need:

• If possible, eliminate the cause (e.g., grass, carpet, etc.).

• Give a daily omega-3 fatty acid supplement with its supportive nutrients. Within 3 weeks allergy symptoms should decrease.

• Add quercetin (p. 131), to the food: small dogs, 100 mg.; medium dogs, 200 mg.; large dogs, 500 mg.

• Add bee pollen to the diet (p. 139).

• Give an antioxidant supplement (pages 41, 43, 45, 46, 117, 118, 119, 121, 138, 144), "whole food," or multiantioxidant formula.

• Add Ester C daily to the diet: small dogs, 100 mg.; medium dogs, 250 mg.; large dogs, 500 mg.

Anemia

If your vet tells you that your dog has anemia, you can do the following:

• Feed a high-quality alternative professional food.

• Provide B vitamin supplements including folic acid, copper and iron, (pages 108–115, 124, 126),

Or use Pet Tinic which contains all the aforementioned vitamins.

• Feed cooked liver three times weekly as an additional meal. Do not add it to your dog's food, because he might not eat it again until you add liver.

Antibiotic Therapy/Intestinal Problems

Successful medical therapy often relies on antibiotics. While alternative therapies are often successful, nothing kills bacteria like an antibiotic. You and your dog have taken plenty throughout your lives, trust me: tetracycline, sulfur, penicillin, just to name a few. The problem is that the antibiotic kills the bad bacteria wherever the infection resides, but it also kills the friendly and necessary bacteria in the intestines. Once enough of the good bacteria are destroyed, your dog will get loose or mucus-coated stools, frequent stools, or diarrhea. Even worse, the intestines can become wounded, allowing everything that your dog puts into his mouth to pass, directly into its bloodstream, bypassing the intestines.

Probiotics, meaning "for life," are the opposite of antibiotics, adding favorable bacteria back to the intestines. These include acidophilus (the fermenting agent in yogurt) and bifida. Since most intestinal problems include a loss of friendly bacteria, probiotics are almost always useful when your dog has intestinal problems such as gas, loose stools with blood or mucus, diarrhea, or constipation. I suggest giving the following:

• Acidophilus in each meal

• B vitamins

• Glutamine

Glutamine is an amino acid that the intestinal cells need for health. Dosage: Large breed type dogs 200 mg. with meals, medium breeds 100 mg. with meals, and small breeds 50 mg. with meals.

Anxiety

Anxiety has many characteristics, including pacing, tremors, excessive biting at a particular area (especially the feet), excessive barking, hiding, poor appetite, and even aggression toward another animal or you. Some dogs become anxious when left alone in the house, when being boarded, just before and during thunderstorms and July 4, when other dogs are around the house, when a new animal or person is brought into the family, changes in routines, and car rides (especially when going to the veterinarian or groomer). To reduce your dog's anxiety, you can do the following:

- Free-feed a moderate quantity of protein food containing a large proportion of wheat and other cereals, without dyes or preservatives.

- Leave honey-sweetened chamomile tea next to the water dish.

- Give Calms Forte homeopathic tablets, available from any health food store: large dogs, adult dose; medium dogs, ½ adult dose; small dogs, child's dose.

- Give B vitamins or brewer's yeast.

- Avoid refined sugar.

- Supplement with magnesium (p. 127).

- Feed warm milk with a dog biscuit.

- Give valerian (p. 144).

Arthritis

Common in older large dogs, long-backed dogs such as dachshunds, small dogs known for knee problems, and after orthopedic surgery, the symptoms of arthritis in dogs are similar to those in humans. Stiffness, limping, problems getting up, crying when the painful areas are touched, and reluctance to run or walk are signs of arthritis. As always, your veterinarian should be the one to diagnose it. To help alleviate the pain and perhaps slow the ongoing progression of this disease, you can do the following:

- Keep the dog in a warm area, sleeping on a water bed or heating pad.

- Encourage small/moderate amounts of exercise.

- Keep his weight normal, feeding a high-quality professional food (diet, if necessary) 3–4 times daily.

- Supplement with alfalfa, a "whole food" antioxidant, (pages 43, 46, 118, 119, 120, 121, 138, 143) or other antioxidant combination.

- Supplement with sea mussels (*Perna canaliculus*) or glucosamine sulfate (available from health food stores or your vet). Dosage for large dogs:

1000 mg., divided, twice daily; medium dogs, 600–800 mg., divided, twice daily; small dogs, 250–500 mg., divided, twice daily.

• Give an omega-3 supplement with supportive nutrients.

• Supplement with Ester C (pages 117–119).

• Supplement with shark cartilage (follow manufacturer's recommended dosage).

• Glucosamine sulfate—dosage for large dogs 500–1000 mg. divided twice daily, medium dogs 250–500 mg. divided twice daily.

Excessive Gas

Once you have experienced the passage of gas by your dog, you will have no problem diagnosing it. The causes can vary from a fast change of food to feeding a food with too many carbohydrates, feeding a food with a fiber that doesn't agree with your dog, fast eating, intestinal worms, too many unfriendly bacteria in the gut, or more serious causes that require your veterinarian's treatment. These include the beginning of bloat, blockage, and intestinal disease. Here are some things you can do:

• Worm the dog, if required; your veterinarian should do this.

• Give charcoal tablets (available at drugstores) at the recommended dosage, after each meal, until gas disappears. Give human dosage for large and giant dogs, ½ for medium-sized dogs and ⅛–¼ for small dogs.

• Change to a home-cooked bland diet (pages 149, 150) or one from your veterinarian. Once the symptoms disappear, slowly introduce a food with a different fiber and less cereal.

• Add probiotics to the food.

• Follow the same methods used for bloat prevention (p. 73).

Cancer Prevention/Post Chemotherapy and Radiation Therapy

A cancer-preventing diet must consist of a high-quality alternative food. If your dog is undergoing treatment for cancer, either with chemo or radiation, it will need a diet high in calories, fat, and protein, and low in carbohydrate. Eukanuba's Prescription Recovery Formula, fed 3–6 times daily, is a good alternative food to serve. Also recommended are the following:

• Supplement with Ester C, (pages 117–119) for prevention and management.

• Supplement with multiantioxidant formula or "natural" whole antioxidant-rich food (pages 43, 44, 45) for prevention and management.

• Add omega-3 fatty acid supplement with balanced nutrients for prevention and management.

• Add brewer's or torula yeast for prevention and management.

• Add shark cartilage at recommended human dosage for large dogs, ½ human dose for medium dogs, and ¼–⅛ human dose for small dogs for prevention. Managing cancer requires higher doses, as directed by your veterinarian

• Do not serve foods, treats, or supplements containing dyes, sodium nitrite, or refined sugars for prevention and management.

• Supplement with acidophilus daily for prevention and management.

• Add a multivitamin–mineral supplement in the form of a "whole food" (bee pollen or wheat grass, pages 45, 47) or a synthetic supplement for prevention and management.

• Add a vegetable enzyme to the food.

Chewing Problems

One of the ways dogs (particularly puppies) relate to the world is by putting things in their mouths. Puppies teethe until their permanent teeth are in place (about 6–9 months). This is the stage where habits develop, right or wrong. Your puppy needs to know that chewing bedroom slippers is unacceptable, but chewing rubber Kong toys or rope toys is okay. You can stuff a hollow long bone or a Kong with peanut butter or cream cheese.

Sometimes, young or old, good habits or bad, dogs become destructive. They tear at the couch, molding, chairs, etc. This is a time to "crate train" your dog, and call a trainer or behaviorist. Crate training means giving your dog security in his own little den, which just happens to be made of aluminum, plastic, or light steel. A crate should be large enough for your dog to sit upright and turn around with ease. The object of crate training is to confine your dog so he cannot be destructive or use any part of your house as a toilet. The crate, soon to be your dog's den, should be made as comfortable as possible; add a pet bed if you want, a few toys, and of course a nonspill water dish and, if your dog eats free-feed, a food dish. If you leave the crate door open and keep it in a room where all the household action is, your dog will likely go in there and just hang out. Once he is used to it, you should keep him in the crate whenever you're not home. If you think he requires toilet relief, have someone walk him during the day. But in the meantime, diet changes should be made (see "Anxiety," p. 51). You can also do the following:

- Replace smaller chunk food with large dry dog food.
- Add a multivitamin–mineral supplement. This is essential.
- Increase the amount of fiber in your dog's food.

Constipation

Hard stools and difficulty passing them are the usual signs of constipation. Older dogs are more prone to it, as are young ones that are fed improperly or have eaten something they shouldn't have. If your dog shows any signs of illness, he must be brought to the veterinarian immediately, since there could be a blockage of the intestinal tract. The following will help your dog:

- Add canned pumpkin to every meal. The dosage can range from ⅛ tsp. for a small dog to ½ tsp. for a large dog, depending on results. Start with ¼ tsp. for medium and large dogs, increasing the amount depending on stool results. Or you can do any of the following:

- Add wheat bran to every meal. Follow same dosages as for pumpkin. For increased taste, combine it with brewer's yeast.

- Put your dog on a high-fiber diet recommended by your veterinarian, changing foods slowly.

- Add water to the food.

- Keep the water dish clean and full of fresh water, to encourage your dog to drink more.

- Supplement with brewer's yeast (p. 47).

- Supplement with acidophilus daily.

- Supplement with folic acid (p. 113).

- Increase the dog's exercise.

- Add vegetable enzyme to the food (p. 145).

Copper Toxicity

Some Breed Dogs such as the West Highland terrier, Bedlington terrier and Portuguese water dog have a genetic fault that can cause abnormal storage of copper in the liver, which can cause liver disease. If your dog is diagnosed with this do the following:

- Feed a diet with no more than 1.2 mg. copper per 100 grams of food.

- Avoid organ meats (liver, kidney).

- Give zinc 3–6 times daily (pages 134–135).
- Feed Hills Prescription Diet Canine I/D™.

Diabetes

Only your vet can diagnose diabetes. Even though the following list is long, all of it is helpful for a diabetic dog. Add one supplement at a time to tolerance, before going on to the next one. Most important, be very, very consistent; feed the same amount of the same food at the same time each day. Your dog must be kept at its proper weight, and exercised moderately every day.

- Use an alternative professional high-quality food only. If your dog is overweight, the diet food must not be supermarket grade. It simply doesn't have enough nutrients and may change ingredients from batch to batch. Purina CNM Brand Veterinary Diet DCO-Formula is an excellent choice.

- Supplement with vegetable enzymes at every meal.

- Add fiber to lower insulin requirements. If your veterinarian has not recommended a food with moderate to high fiber, add oat bran and brewer's yeast to your dog's food: small dogs, ⅛ tsp. oat bran, ⅛ tsp. of brewer's yeast; medium dogs, ¼–½ tsp. oat bran with an equal amount of brewer's yeast; large dogs, ¾ tsp. oat bran and ¾ tsp. brewer's yeast.

- Do not supplement with bee pollen or sugar.

- Supplement with multiple B vitamins.

- Supplement with vitamin C.

- Supplement with chromium which works best when combined with B vitamins. For small dogs, 50 mcg. daily; for medium dogs, 100 mcg. daily; for large dogs, 150–200 mcg. daily. Do not use time-release capsules.

- Add a multivitamin–mineral supplement with calcium, zinc, potassium, and magnesium. Use in treat form or in a "whole natural foods," such as garlic, brewer's yeast, alfalfa, barley or wheatgrass.

Diarrhea or Loose, Watery/Pasty Stools

Because diarrhea can be symptomatic of many different diseases, make sure you have the vet rule out any of them before proceeding to a diet solution. Once given the okay, start by withholding food for 24 hours if the dog is over 6 months old and in relatively good health (don't withhold water).

If your veterinarian does not find a medical reason for this problem, you can resolve it by using the following approach and being extremely patient. A dog's intestines and body require time to readjust.

• Feed a low-residue, easy-to-digest veterinarian intestinal diet or a home-cooked meal 3–6 times daily until the stools start to firm up. Choices of diet include the low residue two-day-only canine diet on page 150, the home-cooked low-residue diet on page 149 for no longer than 10 days, or Prescription Diet I/D (Hills), Eukanuba Low Residue Diet (IAMS), or DCO-formula Canine (Purina). Do not give your dog anything to eat other than his food. That includes rawhide. The two-day low-residue diet is successful only if the problem has just appeared and you can blame it on a simple cause such as anxiety, too many fatty table scraps, cat food, eating garbage, eating old or moldy food, or drinking stagnant, dirty water. If the dog has had this problem for a while, the two-day diet is probably not a good choice because it's doubtful that his intestines will have enough time to get healthy.

If the problem clears up, you can slowly change back to the dog's regular food. If it reappears, then the food is the problem. Change back and keep feeding the veterinary diet, which is low-residue and low-fiber, or you can investigate the ingredients of your prior food and try another with different ingredients but containing low fiber. Since some dogs require more fiber than that found in low residue foods you can do the following:

• Rule out an allergy/sensitivity problem (see p. 49–50).

• Add ⅛–½ tsp. of oat bran plus ⅛–½ tsp. of brewer's yeast, watching stool formation for 2–3 days. If stools begin to normalize, add a little more fiber until they are normal. Or you can do any of the following:

• Add ⅛–1 tsp. of canned pumpkin to your dog's food, increasing the amount depending on the stool consistency.

• Feed a high-fiber diet recommended by your veterinarian.

• Add psyillium powder or Metamucil™ to the diet, starting with a small amount.

• Add a vegetable enzyme (be sure it is not in a lactose base) to the food.

• Supplement with acidophilus daily.

• Avoid foods with sugars or milk.

• Add ¼–1 cup of canned coconut milk to the drinking water or to the food.

Heart Disease

If your dog is suffering from heart disease, the following should be adhered to, after consultation with your vet.

• Smoked or salted foods, shellfish, MSG, processed cheese, carrots, and seaweed are forbidden.

• Feed B vitamins or brewer's yeast.

• Feed Potassium-rich natural foods: brewer's yeast, blackstrap molasses, fresh garlic, dairy, foods, bananas, alfalfa.

• Feed a sodium-restricted food as advised by your veterinarian.

• Have fresh water available at all times.

• If the dog is not on prescription diuretics, add natural ones: chopped cucumbers, dandelion, or parsley.

• If your dog has cardiomyopathy, supplement with L-carnitine.

• Supplement with enzyme.

Hypothyroidism

Your dog's entire body metabolism (heart rate, blood pressure, weight gain or loss, hair growth, muscle usage, etc.) depends upon a normal thyroid gland. If it is not producing enough thyroid hormone, your dog will begin to show symptoms of slow metabolism which include lethargy, hair loss on both sides of the body without itching, weight gain, and scaly skin. The following are helpful:

• Supplement with tyrosine: small dogs, 150 mg.; medium dogs, 250 mg.; large dogs, 500 mg.

• Add seaweed to food daily.

• Supplement with B vitamins.

• Supplement with zinc.

• Supplement with an antioxidant-rich "whole food" or synthetic combination of antioxidants.

• Supplement with selenium.

Kidney Disease

Once upon a time we thought that dogs with kidney disease required a low, but high-quality, protein diet. We now know that in early kidney disease, protein is necessary to help the damaged tissues. DO NOT RESTRICT PROTEIN unless your veterinarian tells you to.

• Feed a high-quality alternative food with moderate (normal) amounts of protein.

• Give omega-3 fatty acid supplements daily.

• Give B vitamin supplements or brewer's yeast daily.

• Potassium is a must: ¼–1 clove of garlic in every meal, or chopped dandelion or blackstrap molasses or a banana a day.

• Restrict calcium and phosphorus.

• Give plenty of fresh water.

• Do not give salty foods.

• Add a fermentable fiber to the food: FOS (Fructooligosaccharides) from the health food store. Follow adult dosage for large dogs, ½ adult dosage for medium dogs, and child's dosage for small dogs.

Liver Disease

If your dog is diagnosed with liver disease, do the following after consultation with your vet:

• Feed a highly digestible food with low or moderate amounts of high-quality protein (ask your veterinarian for the proper food). Feed 3–6 meals daily.

• Any table scraps must consist of high-quality proteins (eggs, cheese, fish).

• Do not feed shellfish or organ meats by-products (liver, kidney, heart).

• Restrict salt.

• Supplement with B vitamins.

• Supplement with vitamin C.

• Do not feed additional fats or fat-soluble vitamins.

• Add a vegetable enzyme to all meals.

• Give acidophilus daily.

Panosteitis

Growing pains is the simplest explanation for this puppy disease. Seen mostly in the larger dogs, the bones are achy when touched, the puppy will limp on either leg or both, and it may not feel like playing. Though genetics may play a role in this, overfeeding is the major culprit, since bones need time to grow slowly and correctly. Overfeeding rushes bone growth and presents problems.

- Slow growth is essential. Don't overfeed or underfeed. Feel for the ribs to determine the correct weight. Keep the puppy on the thin side until 2 years of age.

- Give vitamin C after 1 year of age (p. 116).

- Give B vitamins.

- Feed a high-quality alternative food.

- Don't add supplements other than "natural foods" to the food.

- Do not give additional calcium or bone meal.

- Make sure the dog gets moderate exercise.

- Provide plenty of sunlight.

Shyness

Try one the following remedies at a time, for as long as 1–2 weeks, and monitor the results. If it doesn't work, discontinue it and try the next one.

- Provide him with a safe, cozy area.

- Do not force him to socialize.

- Leave food down all day in a quiet place where your dog feels comfortable.

- Supplement with B vitamins (or brewer's yeast) daily.

- Give Bach Flower Remedies: Aspen, Mimulus, or Rock Rose (available from health food stores). Give adult dosage for large dogs, ½ adult dose for medium dogs, ¼ adult dose for smaller dogs.

- Give Homeopet Anti-Anxiety Drops daily. These are available from Homeopet, (800) 274-7387. Put them directly into the dog's mouth with a medicine dropper or into food.

- Provide a lot of "TLC" and attention with interactive play and regular daily petting and/or brushing. Establish a consistent routine as much as possible. Play at the same place, at same time.

Urinary Tract Problems

The urinary tract consists of the kidneys, ureters, bladder, and urethra. Dogs can get infections and/or develop clumps of sand or stones in any part of the system, usually starting with the bladder. Cystitis concerns only the bladder and is common in dogs. If left untreated and bacterial in origin, the infection can go up to the kidneys. Symptoms include frequent urination (sometimes in inappropriate places because of the extreme need to urinate), reddish-brown urine, darker-than-usual urine, a thick discharge from the penis or vagina, or problems urinating.

• Keep urine acidic (6.2–6.8) rather than basic (except in dalmatians; see below) by feeding foods high in meat and low in cereals. Most alternative high-quality foods produce an acidic urine.

• Have fresh, clean water available at all times.

• Add a pinch of salt to food.

• Add cranberry juice concentrate to food (⅛ tsp. for small dogs, ¼ tsp. for medium dogs, ½ tsp. for large dogs).

• Feed veterinary prescription food for maximum acidity.

• Feed acid-forming foods: asparagus, eggs, fish, meat, milk, pasta.

• Add garlic to the food daily.

• Supplement with vitamin C daily (p. 116).

• Supplement with marshmallow root tincture. Use recommended adult dosage for large breed dogs, ½ adult dose for medium dogs, and child's dose for small dogs.

• Add chopped dandelion or dandelion tea (p. 140) to the food as a supplement.

Note: For some dalmatians, with the appearance of uric acid crystals you'll have to do the following:

• Keep urine basic (7.0–7.5) by feeding foods high in cereal and low in organ meats (heart, liver, kidney).

• Don't add minerals to the diet, since calcium, phosphorus, and magnesium must be reduced.

• Add baking soda to the food: ¼ tsp. per 10 lbs. of body weight.

• Do not feed additional salts or salty foods.

• Feed foods that will produce a basic urine: corn, fruits, molasses, maple syrup, and vegetables.

• Feed the veterinary prescription diet U/D (Hills), but not as a preventive. Not all dalmatians produce uric acid crystals.

Weight Loss: A Diet Plan to Slim and Trim Your Dog

While prevention is best, once you've determined that your dog is overweight, you need to put him on a diet program. While specific breeds have a recommended weight, a weight chart is generally useless because—let's face it—most purebreds don't have perfect conformation and many dogs are a combination of breeds.

IS YOUR DOG OVERWEIGHT?

There are three basic methods to determine if your dog is overweight or not.

• You should be able to feel your dog's ribs, but not see them (coursing breeds are an exception). If there is a slight excess of fat covering the ribs, he's overweight. If the ribs are "buried" under a heavy fat covering, he is obese.

• While standing over your dog, you should see an hourglass figure. That means there is an indentation at the waist from behind the ribs to just before the hips. Breeds differ, but if you can't tell where the waist begins, your dog is too fat.

• Looking at your dog in profile, you should see a stomach tuck beginning just behind the last ribs and going up into the hind legs. If Fido's stomach almost touches the ground, chances are it's time for a weight-loss diet, and certainly more exercise.

Breeds at Risk

While we can't blame it all on breeding, there are breeds that have a greater predisposition for obesity: cocker spaniels, Labrador and golden retrievers, Cairn, West Highland, and Scottish terriers, collies, and chihuahuas.

Neutering

Dog's testicles and ovaries contain a hormone called the "food inhibitory hormone." Once your dog's gonads are removed, so is the hormone that helps to satisfy your dog's hunger. That means that neutered dogs are more likely to overeat than other dogs.

Removal of the gonads also reduces, if not eliminates, the sex drive. Believe it or not, that can slow down the metabolism of a dog, creating obesity if exercise is not incorporated into the daily routine and food is not measured. But don't let the tendency to gain weight stop you from neutering your dog. Exercise and measurement of dog food are necessary for any dog's good health. Although it seems that female dogs are more likely to be overweight than male dogs, hormones can't take all the blame. Let's admit it; dog owners cause obesity.

HEALTHY WEIGHT MAINTENANCE PROGRAM

If the weight evaluation above determined that your dog is the correct weight, mark it on the calendar and health records for reference. This evaluation should be performed monthly.

• Feed an alternative high-quality food. If your dog is not overweight, follow recommended feeding directions. If he is overweight, reduce the amount by 25%.

• If you're feeding a "lite" dog food (alternative or supermarket) with fat below 4% and/or fiber above 4%, supplementation is necessary. Supplementation with a vegetable enzyme will help ensure that most, if not all, the fat gets delivered into the body. While low-fat food will help dogs lose weight, it can jeopardize the immune system, and the skin and coat, creating flaky skin and a dull, brittle coat. The addition of a fatty acid supplement can be useful, providing you use the minimum amount so that the fat in the supplement doesn't add too many calories to the food. If the "lite dog food" contains over 4% fiber, unless that fiber happens to be beet pulp, rice bran, or tomato pomace, the addition of acidophilus and/or FOS is necessary to keep the intestinal cells healthy. FOS is a carbohydrate that produces friendly bacteria like acidophilus once it is broken down in the intestines. My favorite light dog foods are Eukanuba

Light (Iams), Eukanuba Veterinary Diets Restricted Calorie, and Veterinary Diet CNM GL Formula.

• Feed at least twice daily if there is no weight problem. Overweight dogs need to be fed 3–6 times daily. Make sure that you don't exceed the quantity of food you are supposed to feed daily. Measure every meal. Every time your dog smells and eats food, believe it or not, he burns some calories!

• No table scraps or treats allowed! Fool your dog by putting his dog food where the treats are kept, and give him his dog food. Don't forget to deduct that amount from his total daily quantity (already measured).

• Reward with love or exercise rather than food.

• Exercise your dog at least twice daily—20 mins. each time is optimum. If your dog isn't used to exercise, start out on a mild program and increase the level of activity gradually.

• Monitor your dog's weight weekly.

DR. JANE'S WEIGHT LOSS PROGRAM FOR OVERWEIGHT DOGS

If your evaluation determined that your dog doesn't have a waistline or detectable ribs, this program is for him. Although some dog owners believe that canine weight loss is difficult, it's not when it's part of an overall health program that combines exercise and grooming with a healthy diet and the appropriate supplements.

To start this healthy program, record your dog's weight and weigh him weekly, marking it on the calendar. Weight loss must be slow: no more than 1 lb. weekly for a large dog; 1 lb. every 2–3 weeks or monthly for medium dogs; and 1 lb. monthly for small dogs. Fast weight reduction not only doesn't work, it is harmful to your dog. Follow the program until the desired weight has been reached.

Before You Begin

Consult your veterinarian and have him give your dog a thorough checkup before you begin this program. This checkup should include a thyroid test. Since portion-controlled feeding is essential for weight loss, free-feeding is out and free-feeding portion-control or mealtime is in.

You need to determine your dog's total daily amount of food requirement and divide it by the number of meals you will feed per day. The quantity of food can be determined by calories (use formula in chapter 2, p. 29) or recommended feeding directions from the can or bag. I would like you to follow the suggested calories or amount of food required for a normal dog. If there is little or no weight loss after a month, then you may decrease the amount you feed by 25%. Thus, if you determine that your dog should be fed 3 cups daily, and you feed or fill the dish three times a day, each meal will consist of 1 cup. Do not exceed total daily rec-ommendation. If your dog still doesn't lose weight with the 25% decrease in food, then you need to change to a diet food. I prefer an alternative professional one.

An important component of this weight loss program involves supple-mentation. For those owners who are feeding dry food only, you have the following options:

a. Sprinkle water onto the food, moistening the nuggets just enough to allow powders to stick. If he doesn't seem to enjoy his food as before, that's a bonus.

b. Add a small amount of garlic powder, or desiccated powdered liver combined with the supplement, to the food, plus just enough water to mix. The bonus—health benefits from the garlic and liver.

c. Add a small amount of canned food from the same manufacturer. If one is not available, add a supermarket canned food to an alternative pro-fessional dry food. Quantities: small dogs ⅛ tsp. of canned food plus enough water to make a gravy; medium dogs, ¼–½ teaspoon; large dogs, no more than one teaspoon.

You'll note that in the program, I recommend *Garcinia cambogia* (see p. 142) in capsule form. It is often marketed under the brand name Citra-max™. Open the capsule and pour the recommended amount onto food or put the capsule directly into your dog's mouth, if you can. I also recom-mend a multivitamin–mineral treat, and you must get one that contains fatty acids. Other general notes about the program: I've indicated with an asterisk (*) which choice is preferred when there is more than one; and the times for play and toilet necessities can be changed to conform to your schedule. Also, when I say to add 3 additional minutes to a walk time, the goal is to get to at least a 20-minute walk for each walk of the day. Your overweight dog may not be able to do that much at first, so you have to build up to it. Now let's begin the program.

Sunday

Goals: Exercise and grooming.

Morning

Post-Potty Reward: Multivitamin–mineral treat.

Exercise #1: *Garcinia cambogia* in pill form (optional). Walk at least 3 mins. more than usual.

Water: Add Norwegian sea kelp (optional) to the water: 1 drop for small dog, 2 drops for medium, 3 drops for large.

Breakfast: Morning portion of dog food. Supplement with *Garcinia cambogia* (Citramax powder), if not given earlier, and fresh garlic.

Sunday Play: No earlier than 1 hr. after eating, play a game, such as catch, Frisbee™, tug-of-war, hide-and-seek, etc. Length of time depends on Fido's condition. Don't be ashamed to limit play to 5 mins. Optimum length is 20 mins.-plus.

Home-Alone Treat: ¼–2 cups of plain popcorn, given one by one or as a snack; ¼–2 cups of raw diced zucchini or broccoli, plus rawhide or cow ear or hoof.

Late Afternoon/After Work

Post-Potty Reward: Diced cucumber* or celery.

Exercise #2: Usual walk time with 3 additional mins. minimum.

Lunch: Afternoon portion of dog food plus ¼ tsp.–¼ cup of chopped fresh* or dry parsley, or dandelion. If you have the time, you can make this home-cooked meal, beef and vegetable medley, as a substitute:

⅛–½ lb. chopped lean meat	1 tbsp.–¼ c. chopped raw or cooked
Vegetable oil	vegetables (broccoli)*
1 egg	Fresh garlic to taste

Pour just enough oil to cover the bottom of the pan. Sauté garlic, then add meat and vegetables. Stir in beaten egg. Remove from heat once meat turns brown. Bring to room temperature and serve.

Post-Potty Reward: Carrots or celery.

Exercise #3 (optional): Usual walk, with 3 additional mins.

Grooming Time: Bathe or brush; tail to head and head to tail.

Treat: Chew toy.

Evening

Water: Refill water dish if necessary.

Dinner: Evening portion of dog food plus fresh garlic, brewer's yeast, kelp (if not added to water earlier).

Post-Potty Reward: Diced apples.

Exercise #3 or #4: Usual walk, with 3 additional mins.

Bedtime Treat: ¼–2 cups of cooked vegetables, 1 cup dandelion tea (optional).

Monday

Goal: Clean ears and eyes.

Post-Potty Reward: Multivitamin–mineral treat.

Exercise #1: Usual walk, same length as Sunday. Give *Garcinia cambogia* in pill form (optional).

Water: Clean water bowl. Add fresh water and kelp (optional; can be added to the food).

Breakfast: Morning portion of dog food, plus *Garcinia cambogia*, if not given earlier, plus fresh garlic.

Home-Alone Treat: Marrow bone plus ½–2 cups of plain popcorn (optional).

Late Afternoon/After Work
Post-Potty Reward: Slices of cucumber* or carrots.

Exercise #2: Usual walk, *Garcinia cambogia* in pill form (optional).

Water: Add more water if necessary.

Lunch: Second portion of dog food, plus ¼ tsp.–¼ cup of chopped parsley or dandelion.

Treat: Individual pieces of popcorn to satisfy begging, and any type of chew toy.

Evening
Water: Refill bowl if necessary.

Dinner: Evening portion of dog food, plus fresh garlic, brewer's yeast, Norwegian kelp (if not given earlier).

Post-Potty Reward: Sliced carrots.

Exercise #3: Usual walk.

Bedtime Treat: Clean ears and eyes; love; give marrow bone or toy.

Tuesday

Goal: Clean teeth and lots of TLC.

Morning
Post-Potty Reward: Multivitamin–mineral treat.

Exercise #1: Usual walk plus 3 mins., *Garcinia cambogia* in pill form (optional).

Water: Clean water bowl. Add fresh water and kelp (optional; can be added to the food).

Breakfast: Morning portion of dog food, *Garcinia cambogia* (if not given earlier), fresh garlic.

Home-Alone Treat: Chew toy plus ½–3 cups of plain popcorn (optional).

Late Afternoon/After Work

Post-Potty Reward: Sliced apple or cucumber*.

Exercise #2: Usual walk, same length as morning; *Garcinia cambogia*, in pill form (optional).

Water: Add more water if necessary.

Lunch: Second portion of dog food plus ¼ tsp.–¼ cup chopped parsley or dandelion.

Treat: Individual pieces of popcorn to satisfy begging, plus one chew toy.

Evening

Water: Refill bowl if necessary.

Dinner: Evening portion of dog food plus fresh garlic, brewer's yeast, and kelp (if not given earlier).

Post-Potty Reward: Piece of celery.

Exercise #3: Usual walk, same length as morning.

Bedtime: Clean teeth; love; give chew toy.

Wednesday

Goal: Brush and comb.

Morning

Post-Potty Reward: Multivitamin–mineral treat.

Exercise #1: Usual walk plus 3 mins. more, *Garcinia cambogia*, in pill form (optional).

Water: Clean water bowl. Add kelp to fresh water (optional; can be added to the food later).

Breakfast: Morning portion of dog food, plus *Garcinia cambogia*, if not given earlier, plus fresh garlic.

Home-Alone Treat: Chew toy plus ½–3 cups of popcorn.

Late Afternoon/After Work

Post-Potty Reward: Slices of cucumber* or zucchini.

Exercise #2: Usual walk plus 3 mins., *Garcinia cambogia* in pill form (optional).

Water: Refill water bowl.

Lunch: Second portion of dog food, plus ¼ tsp.–¼ cup chopped parsley or dandelion.

Treat: Broken bits of brown rice cakes to satisfy begging, and chew toy.

Evening

Water: Refill bowl if necessary.

Dinner: Evening portion of dog food plus fresh garlic, Norwegian kelp (if not given earlier), and brewer's yeast.

Post-Potty Reward: Sliced carrot or apple.

Exercise #3: Usual walk.

Bedtime: Brush, comb, and love; give chew toy.

Thursday

Goal: Clean teeth.

Morning

Post-Potty Reward: Multivitamin–mineral treat.

Exercise #1: Usual walk plus 3 additional mins., *Garcinia cambogia* in pill form.

Water: Clean bowl. Add kelp to fresh water (optional; can be added to food later).

Breakfast: Morning portion of dog food, *Garcinia cambogia* (if not given earlier), and fresh garlic.

Home-Alone Treat: Chew toy plus ½–3 cups of plain popcorn (optional).

Late Afternoon/After Work

Post-Potty Reward: Pieces of carrot or cucumber*.

Exercise #2: Usual walk, *Garcinia cambogia* (optional).

Water: Add fresh water to bowl.

Lunch: Second portion of dog food plus ¼ tsp.–¼ cup chopped parsley.

Treat: Pieces of fennel* or celery to satisfy begging, plus one chew toy.

Evening

Water: Refill the bowl if necessary.

Dinner: Evening portion of dog food plus fresh garlic, Norwegian kelp (if not added earlier), and brewer's yeast.

Post-Potty Reward: Pieces of fennel* or celery.

Exercise #3: Usual walk.

Bedtime: Clean teeth; love; give chew toy.

Friday

Goal: Increase exercise with additional play time.

Morning

Post-Potty Reward: Pieces of fennel* or cucumber.

Exercise #1: Usual walk plus 3 mins., *Garcinia cambogia* in pill form (optional).

Water: Clean water bowl. Add fresh water and kelp (optional; can be added to the food).

Breakfast: Morning portion of dog food, plus *Garcinia cambogia* (if not given earlier) and fresh garlic.

Home-Alone Treat: Chew toy.

Late Afternoon/After Work

Post-Potty Reward: Pieces of zucchini* or other vegetable.

Exercise #2: Usual walk, *Garcinia cambogia* (optional).

TGIF Play Time: Tug-of-war, fetch, frisbee.

Water: Add more water to bowl if needed.

Lunch: Second portion of dog food, plus ¼ tsp.–¼ cup chopped parsley.

Treat: Pieces of fennel* or apple.

Evening

Water: Refill bowl with fresh water.

Dinner: Evening portion of dog food, fresh garlic, Norwegian kelp (if not given earlier), and brewer's yeast.

Post-Potty Reward: Pieces of apple.

Exercise #3: Walk.

Bedtime: Love, dandelion tea, and chew toy.

Saturday

Goal: Clean ears and eyes; another play session.

Morning

Post-Potty Reward: Multivitamin–mineral treat.

Exercise #1: Usual walk plus 5 mins., *Garcinia cambogia* in pill form (optional).

Waters: Clean water bowl. Add fresh water and kelp (optional; can be added to the food).

Breakfast: Morning portion of dog food, *Garcinia cambogia* (if not given earlier), fresh garlic.

Treat: ¼–2 cups cooked spinach and/or ¼–2 cups of popcorn.

Afternoon

Post-Potty Reward: Diced cucumber.

Exercise #2: Usual walk, plus *Garcinia cambogia* (optional).

Lunch: Afternoon portion of dog food, plus ¼ tsp.–¼ cup of chopped fresh dandelion or parsley.

Water: Add fresh water to bowl if needed.

Play Session: Interactive game (your choice), minimum 5 mins., 20 mins. optimum.

Treat: Marrow bone or chew toy.

Evening

Water: Add fresh water to bowl.

Dinner: Evening portion of dog food, plus fresh garlic, brewer's yeast, and kelp (if not added to water).

Post-Potty Reward: Vegetable of your choice.

Bedtime: Treat (1–3 hard-boiled or soft-boiled eggs) and love.

CHAPTER SIX

Special Needs of Special Breeds

I don't care what anyone says, dogs are not all the same! They were the first animal to be domesticated during the Stone Age; their amazing variety in size, shape, color, and personality has produced, to date, 134 AKC-recognized breeds. While the first *Canis lupus familiaris* weighed about 30–40 pounds, and was colored to blend in with the flora of the period, today's breeds can range from as little as 3 pounds for a Chihuahua to 210 pounds for an Irish wolfhound or Great Dane. Depending on the size of the dog, the amount of coat and its texture, skin type, eye formation, size of nose, generalized form, country of origin, and of course personality, breeds will have their own special dietary needs.

While this chapter can't include EVERY breed registered with the AKC, and others, I've selected the more popular breeds and will discuss their particular problems, how to avoid them, and what to do about them. If you have a mixed breed, or if your breed is not discussed in this chapter, look up the breed(s) that most closely resembles your dog. If your dog doesn't fit my abbreviated description and problems, realize that all dogs have their own unique personalities and nuances, and that your dog is one of a kind!

Bloat

Simply stated, bloat is a digestion related trauma that can lead to death. It occurs most often in large and giant dogs or deep-chested dogs, but can occur in other breeds. This complex disease consists of one or more components. First the stomach fills with gas and expands. A dog with this first component will belch, pass wind, vomit, and be unsettled due to the discomfort. The gas-filled stomach can then twist, cutting off circulation to the stomach and creating a life-threatening trauma.

Causes: Genetic predisposition; overeating; fast eating, which results in gulping air; exercise on a full stomach; too much water at one time; calcium supplementation, which causes the stomach to empty slower than usual.

Prevention: Don't supplement with calcium. Free-feed portion-control or at least two meals daily. Feed a high-quality food so that the quantity is limited. No physical activity until at least an hour after meals. Give access to fresh water at all times. No competitive feeding. Feed dogs from dishes that are shoulder height so that they don't have to raise and lower their heads, which increases the amount of air they consume.

Common myths: It was once thought that foods containing a high quantity of cereal, including soy, created bloat because of the fermentation. It was also thought that dry food expands in the stomach, so moistening it or feeding canned was better.

HOUND GROUP

Afghan Hound

An elegant athlete, this beautiful dog takes pride in its long, flowing, silky coat. A coat that is dull, sparse, short, or feels like cotton is unacceptable. A high-quality alternative professional food is a must. Brewer's yeast or spirulina treats can be a plus. Bloat prevention (see sidebar) is a good idea. Vegetable enzymes are a must because they will ensure better digestion (for bloat prevention) and nutrient delivery to the coat. Since well-developed muscles, healthy lungs, and a strong heart are assets during field trials, the addition of L-carnitine- and taurine-rich foods (wheat germ, torula yeast, raw meat) makes good sense.

American Foxhound

A muscular, deep-chested dog with floppy ears, his nutritional requirements are a combination of all the other hounds: bloat prevention (see sidebar), brewers yeast and garlic, and vegetable-, or L-carnitine- and taurine-rich treat supplements. Since a thin, short coat is an obvious fault, a high-quality food or a supermarket food plus a vegetable enzyme is advisable.

Basenji

A truly ancient breed. While its skin and coat may not require much care, the basenji certainly requires attention and play. It is easily bored, so leaving dry food down all day can help satisfy it. No need to worry about calories, since this dog doesn't gain weight easily. A hollow bone stuffed with peanut butter helps to make the day go by faster.

Basset Hound

These gentle, fearless dogs make wonderful guardians, but need some special care. Their skin can become a battleground for all types of skin disease. A high-quality professional diet is essential. A daily supplementation of bee pollen or spirulina will provide some of the immune-boosting nutrients they require. Bloat prevention (see p. 73) is a must because of their deep chests. They are prone to arthritis, so antioxidants after 2 years of age are a necessary preventive. Carrots and celery are excellent treats that will add fiber but not calories. It's difficult enough to get a basset hound to do what you want it to do without its being fat!

🐾 Frisbee™-Playing

Definition: Throwing a disk of any material (soft or hard) into the air for a dog to retrieve, preferably in midair.

Pros: Great general exercise for the dog with little exertion by the owner; increases motor skills of the dog; strengthens thigh and chest muscles; great fun for training.

Cons: Because it involves muscles, tendons, and ligaments of the hips, in young large/giant breeds this kind of activity can "loosen" the newly developing joint structure, which develops very slowly in them. I require a dog to be at least 18 months old prior to jumping.

Beagle

Big brown eyes, floppy ears, and a desire to please its owner make the beagle America's favorite dog. While beagles may tend to bark a little too much, they are certainly easy to care for as long as you remember to clean the ears 3–4 times a week and brush their coat daily, distributing the oils throughout. Beagles seem to do well on all types of food, as long as it's not in abundance. If dandruff becomes an issue, change to a better-quality food with a higher-quality protein and add a hard-or soft-boiled egg daily, or feed a fatty acid treat.

Bloodhound

Who can't love those big eyes, long ears, and loving personality? The best way to keep their skin, ears, and joints healthy is to feed a high-quality alternative professional food in a dish elevated to shoulder height, and to keep the 2 or 3 meals on the skimpy side rather than overfeeding. Since bloat is a real problem in this breed, a vegetable enzyme should be added to the food to ensure increased digestion. (See bloat prevention p. 73). Washing the ears with equal parts vinegar and water 3–4 times a week is imperative to keep them clean. Their average life span is under 10 years, so antioxidants after the age of 2 are essential.

Borzoi Russian Wolfhound

Elegant, big, and sweet, this dog is truly extraordinary. It is plagued with the same problems as other large dogs: bloat, hip dysplasia, and cardiomyopathy. Bloat prevention (see p. 73) and the addition of L-carnitine- and taurine-rich foods (torula yeast, raw meat, wheat germ) are absolute musts. While genetics, grooming, and a high-quality alternative professional food will help ensure a luxurious coat, a skin and coat supplement in the form of a treat is a great idea. Life extension is important for these giants, so antioxidants as either a supplement or a treat are a must for any dog over 2 years of age.

Coonhound

Adored for his agility, power, and alertness, he is a gentle dog that just doesn't give up. He looks his best with well-exercised muscles and a shiny coat without dander or oil. Brewer's yeast and garlic are the perfect treats or supplements for this dog; they give the skin and coat protein and support nutrients while boosting the immune system to help prevent infections in his floppy ears. An oily coat may require additional vitamin E, so you may as well supplement with a multiantioxidant formula. If you're working the dog, L-carnitine- and taurine-rich foods (wheat germ, torula yeast, raw meat) make good sense.

Dachshunds

Wire-haired, smooth, or long-haired, miniature or regular, these large dogs in a small dog's body are one of my favorites. Obesity can make this little "hot dog" look and feel anything but handsome. Since back and knee problems often occur as they age, biscuits should be discouraged even at a young age. Carrots and celery are excellent treats, and daily antioxidants are also necessary.

English Foxhound

Though stouter than his American cousin, he requires the same nutritional aids as the other hounds. Calorie-counting and exercise are a must for the older dog, because an overweight foxhound just isn't socially acceptable!

Greyhound

Eager to please, not subject to boredom when the owner is away, this gentle giant can make the perfect pet. Its coat and skin need little work except for daily brushing and a well-balanced diet with good-quality protein. Brewer's yeast treats can help ensure adequate protein for strong muscle development and a healthy skin and coat. Carrots, celery, and other vegetables are other treats of choice to keep your greyhound fashionably trim. Because of its large size, bloat, cardiomyopathy, and arthritis are the major diseases to look for and avoid. Take care to prevent bloat (see p. 73. The addition of fresh meat, torula yeast, or wheat germ is a heart saver, since they contain high quantities of L-carnitine and taurine. Antioxidants (alfalfa preferred in this case) are a must for all greyhounds over 2 years of age to help prevent or decrease pain and stiffness.

Harrier

This breed looks much like a smaller edition of the American foxhound, and has the same requirements.

Ibizan Hound

This elegant, short-haired or wire-haired dog, dating back to the Egyptian pharaohs, resembles a greyhound, and thus has the nutritional requirements of one.

Irish Wolfhound

Huge, proud, strong dogs, they deserve responsible owners who can deal with their potential problems of bloat (see p. 73), hip dysplasia, and heart disease. Antioxidants are essential, but I wouldn't use vitamin C until after 2 years of age, to make sure that nothing interferes with the development of the long bones. A high-quality professional food is your only option because bone growth is a must. Exercise will develop those wonderful muscles and help control weight. No Frisbee™ until 2 years of age.

Norwegian Elkhounds

This gray, hardy, dense-coated dog is known for its endurance. If you don't want a dog that sheds, or requires long, brisk walks, perhaps you should stay away from this breed. If you're feeding a supermarket food, a vegetable enzyme or a skin and coat supplement, such as brewer's yeast and garlic or a fatty acid supplement, will help improve the coat and decrease shedding. Since I can't imagine putting flea powder through this coat, brewer's yeast and garlic is a good choice treat or supplement to help repel fleas while keeping the coat at its best.

Otterhound

This rough, tough dog looks like a combination of terrier and hound, with webbed feet. His coat is thick, curly, and oily, which is perfect for the swimming that he loves. A professional alternative food is as important as daily exercise. With the dense outer coat and water-resistant undercoat, brewer's yeast and garlic is a must for a healthy coat and fewer fleas. Since excessively oily skin can be a problem, vitamin E or a combination antioxidant with E may be required.

Petit Basset Griffon Vendeen

This small French hound is noted for its mental and physical stamina as well as its rough, long coat. A high-quality protein food helps him reach his full mental and physical potential. Floppy ears and the long, thick coat makes this dog a candidate for brewer's yeast and garlic supplements, perfect for training this bright little dog. If he gets too excited at times, a natural antianxiety supplement (p. 51) may be helpful.

Pharaoh Hound

Said to be one of the oldest domesticated dogs in recorded history, it is similar to the other large, smooth-haired hounds, and thus has similar nutritional requirements. Since its beautiful amber eyes are one of its greatest assets, deter cataracts by starting antioxidants at 2 years of age.

Rhodesian Ridgeback

Determined watchdogs, these muscled animals need exercise, high-quality food, and love. Because they can manifest the same problems as any big dog—bloat (see p. 73) and hip dysplasia—precautions must be taken. Skin and coat supplements can add that shine your dog may lack, but go easy on the oils because calories count.

Saluki

The royal dog of Egypt is perhaps the oldest known breed of domesticated dog. With muscles made for tremendous speed and and a strong constitution, this elegant dog needs no pampering. To ensure an elegant coat, an alternative professional food should be fed. Take all the bloat precautions (see p. 73) seriously. Since daily antioxidants are life extenders, supplements can be started after the age of 2, or the addition of wheat, oat, or barley grass can begin with puppy food.

Scottish Deerhound

A giant of a dog, this breed has all the requirements of every hound (except supplementation with vitamin E). L-carnitine- and taurine-rich foods are a must, as are antioxidants to help extend his life span.

Whippet

Sometimes thought of as a miniature greyhound, this small hound needs a high-quality food so it can develop the muscular body it's so well known for. Daily exercise is a must for these natural athletes, even if it's just a walk around the block. High-quality protein is the key to good nutrition, and overfeeding is to be avoided.

TERRIER GROUP

Airedales

A breed of dog that's tough and fast enough to hunt leopards, yet gentle enough to be trained as rescue dogs. Develop and maintain that stamina with high-quality protein and high-quality fat. Daily brushing can go a long way for this breed, both for looks and for bonding. If your young bonding partner is a little too active for you, give him some chamomile tea or warm milk with a biscuit before company arrives or before bed.

American Staffordshire Terrier

This muscular Mack truck makes a wonderful companion. Because of their need to chew, make sure that Nylabones™, Kong toys, and other nondestructible items are readily available. A large meat bone, absolutely too big to be swallowed, will clean his teeth and satisfy his need to chew. Leaving your dog's food available all day (not to exceed manufacturer's recommended daily amount) may decrease his hunger so he chews his food and cleans his teeth. Brewer's yeast with garlic will help keep the skin and coat healthy-looking.

Australian Terrier

This rough-coated, compact dog is one of the smallest working terriers. A supermarket food plus vegetable enzymes should be fine if you are not showing him. Because he never tires, the supermarket food, generally higher in cereal, may be enough to slow him down a little. If it isn't, natural antianxiety supplements may be required. Kong toys, bones stuffed with peanut butter, and toys like the Buster cubes are essential. Exercise is vital.

Bedlington Terrier

As cute and resilient as these dogs can look, a lurking copper storage disease can be lethal. Copper quantities vary among foods, so the lower the better, but note that this dog's magnificent sheeplike coat requires a high-quality protein and fat food. (No copper restriction unless your veterinarian says so.) He is prone to some nervousness; chamomile tea calms nerves or an upset stomach.

Border Terrier

The true English farm working dog, this breed loves to work and, like other terriers, often behaves better on supermarket foods, with the addition of vegetable enzymes to help the development of the muscles and all-around health. Exercise is vital.

Bull Terrier

This strong, muscular, active, and intelligent animal requires exercise to keep mind and body well. High-quality protein and fat are an absolute must. Keeping them occupied during your absence requires hollow bones filled with peanut butter, nondestructible chew toys, and any interactive toy you can design. Hang a strong spring from the doorway and tie a rope to it that's just long enough for the dog to reach when he jumps up. Connect a hard rubber toy to the rope. If shedding becomes a problem, a fatty acid skin and coat supplement or vegetable enzymes are needed.

Cairn Terriers

Toto in *The Wizard of Oz* made this breed famous. These "hard coated" dogs develop the best wiry outer coat and thick, soft undercoat on a high-quality protein and fat food. Shedding can become a problem, so in order to increase the nutrient uptake from the good food you are feeding, vegetable enzymes are recommended. If their love of cold weather and snow necessitates frequent baths, add a fatty acid skin and coat conditioner to the diet or as a treat. While their high energy level doesn't make them candidates for diets, carrots and celery are better treats than biscuits.

Dandie Dinmont Terrier

Bloat prevention (see p. 73) is wise for this deep-chested, fast-moving terrier. His rough, double coat makes him the perfect candidate for brewer's yeast and garlic, particularly during the summer. Since the hair can tend to matt, a good-quality food is necessary. Vegetable enzymes can be added to that food if necessary.

Fox Terrier

Whether yours has a smooth coat or a wire coat, his personality is pleasant. If he could smile, he would. While you wouldn't think that this dog requires more than an average food, shedding can be a problem, so feed a high-quality protein and fat food. Adding a vegetable enzyme supplement (p. 145) will deliver the extra nutrients needed. Plenty of exercise and interactive play and toys are critical to these dogs.

Irish Terrier

A well-muscled, sturdy breed, this "clown" requires toys, lots of play time, and portion-controlled feedings. If his stomach is always full, he may be a tad more mannerly, especially when the children are home with him. Supermarket food can be fed, but add a vegetable enzyme to increase the amount of nutrition your dog gets from the food.

Jack Russell Terrier

These active little dogs' strong leg and chest muscles need a high-quality protein food with high-quality fat. Whether smooth- or wire-coated, these dogs require little fuss. For an added boost, add bee pollen to their food daily.

Kerry Blue Terrier

This dog does everything well, from herding sheep to hunting, retrieving, and K9 police work! They are known to be long-lived, and antioxidants will help ensure that. They are stately dogs known for strong muscles and dense, wavy hair, both of which need high-quality alternative food and brewer's yeast and garlic for summer flea control and general coat maintenance.

Lakeland terrier

A dense-coated dog like the Kerry blue, he should be fed a high-quality professional food to maximize his dense, weather-resistant coat. If the skin becomes oily, supplement with an antioxidant containing vitamin E.

Manchester Terrier

This small, intelligent dog with a body that could resemble a hound's, is easy to care for. If you're feeding supermarket food, add vegetable enzymes. Owners tend to make this streamlined dog too fat. He needs portion-controlled free-feeding with vegetable treats only.

Miniature Bull Terrier

Believe it or not, a 16-pound bull terrier has the same nutritional requirements as the big one. Vegetable treats please; he can get too fat.

Miniature Schnauzer

This dog with a stocky build, wiry coat, and abundant whiskers and feathers on its legs needs an alternative quality food to him in top shape. Don't forget to wipe his whiskers after eating.

Norfolk Terrier

This small little dog is very similar to the Norwich; both are known for their muscular thighs, compact body, and protective, hard, wiry coat. Supermarket food, which generally has a high quantity of cereal, plus vegetable enzymes, constitutes the food of choice. If fed portion-controlled free-choice, your terrier should save his energy until you want to play.

Norwich Terrier

See *Norfolk Terrier.*

Sealyham Terrier

If given exercise, a balanced diet (supermarket or alternative), antioxidants after 2 years of age, and love, this dog should live up to its reputation for a long life.

Scottish Terriers

Muscles, coat, and personality are the big three for this alert, lovable, but independent dog. High-quality protein with good-quality fat is essential for this "hard coat" breed with its wiry outer coat and soft, thick undercoat. Brewer's yeast or spirulina would make a great treat. Omega-3 fatty acids should be used to reduce the severe biting and scratching that all too often plague this breed. Because liver problems are common, add a small amount of cooked liver to the food 3 times weekly for protection. Lixotinic is a liver tonic available through your veterinarian for dogs that require concentrated liver support nutrients.

Skye Terrier

This elegant dog has a coat any other dog would envy. A high-quality alternative professional food is a must to keep this coat sleek. The addition of a vegetable enzyme with spirulina or brewer's yeast and garlic treats is a plus.

Staffordshire Bull Terrier

This stout dog is remarkable-looking when he's kept at his best: shiny coat, no dandruff, and well-built muscles. An alternative high-quality food, frequent brushing, and exercise will make you a proud owner. Non-destructible chew toys are essential because they love to chew.

Welsh Terrier

This breed is known for his sturdy, compact, rugged-looking body with a wired coat. High-quality protein food and exercise are essential for muscle development. His dense coat requires frequent brushing so that the oils from the skin can be distributed through the hair. Since he can be a little too spirited at times, portion-controlled free-feeding is a must, and a natural antianxiety supplement from time to time can be a relief.

West Highland White Terrier

This package of spunk, determination, and love is not without its problems. To ensure a healthy skin and coat, a high-quality protein and fat diet is essential, coupled with a brewer's yeast and garlic supplement or treat. Cooked liver twice weekly will supply additional B vitamins. Since they love to play and please you, reward them with a spirulina or antioxidant treat. They are prone to allergies, so bee pollen should be added to their food.

Wheaten Terriers

This smart, affectionate, gentle watchdog thinks he owns you! Whether wire- or soft-coated, he should be fed a professional alternative dry food, left down all day. The good-quality protein and high fat will help keep either type of coat in good condition, and nibbling during the day should help keep energy levels calmer. Brewer's yeast and garlic are wonderful skin and coat treats. Allergies can be a real problem in this breed, so early weaning is not recommended, and altering the diet every 3–5 months (changing slowly, with acidophilus supplemention) may be helpful. Bee pollen will help keep the immune system in check, and try to stay away from highly allergic foods: corn, milk, soy, and eggs. Since this breed suffers from intestinal and kidney disease, any abnormality in stool or urine should be brought to the attention of a veterinarian immediately. Don't assume that loose stool is due to poor eating habits.

WORKING GROUP

Akita

This strong, cuddly, affectionate, protective dog can make the perfect pet, providing it's cared for properly. Daily brushing, combined with a high-quality protein and fat food with vegetable enzymes, will keep the skin and coat healthy, with less shedding. Akitas are prone to obesity, often concealed by the full coat, so carrots and celery are the only treats allowed except for brewer's yeast and garlic for flea control, and skin and coat health. The daily addition of alfalfa provides antioxidants in the food and supports normal bone growth.

Alaskan Malamute

Affectionate, friendly dogs, malamutes need to be worked, or else boredom sets in and your house will pay the price. Because they are picky eaters, leave down a high-quality protein and fat food so they will have the entire day to met their nutritional needs while keeping their stomachs full. Vegetable enzymes added to the food, along with daily combing and brushing, are essential to decrease shedding. If you're feeding a supermarket food, add bee pollen plus a fatty acid supplement. Brewer's yeast and garlic are welcome skin and coat treats, especially during flea season.

Bermese Mountain Dog

This sturdy breed has the same nutritional requirements as the Saint Bernard.

Bull Mastiff

Talk about a big, stout dog! Bloat prevention (see p. 73), slow growth for healthy bones and muscles, an alternative professional food, and exercise are all required. If the coat gets brittle, add a fatty acid supplement.

Boxer

Sometimes you wonder if a clown isn't hiding under all that muscle and muzzle. Exercise and a high-quality protein and fat food are musts. If necessary during the winter, add a fatty acid coat and skin supplement. Since cancer seems to be more common in this breed, the addition of wheat or barley grass or another antioxidant is essential.

Doberman

Intelligent, loyal, and dedicated, this breed is not without its physical problems. Skin disease is common in all Dobermans, particularly blue ones. A quality alternative food is a must, supplemented with vegetable enzymes and bee pollen, algae, or spirulina. Dandruff is not necessarily from dry skin, so before you start adding a fatty acid supplement, check to see if your Doberman, like many, is hypothyroid. If that is the case, you want your supplement to contain kelp or sea algae. As with any skin problem, brewer's yeast and garlic is the treat of choice. Just in case your Doberman is a candidate for Van Willebrand's disease, add liver to its diet or feed liver treats at least once weekly. If anemia is a problem, Pet Tinic is a good supplement.

Great Dane

This giant dog needs a lot of preventive care, starting when it's a puppy. Bloat prevention (see p. 73), is necessary, and no exercise until an hour after eating, and no Frisbee™ or jumping exercises until his joints are well established at 2 years of age; all very important. Keeping the puppy on the thin side is mandatory. Supply antioxidants beginning in puppyhood, with the addition of alfalfa, oat, or barley grass to the high-quality food you need to feed. A vegetable enzyme is also a good idea. Dry food, portion-controlled should be your choice, since canned food simply tastes too good. Because of the potential for heart disease, L-carnitine- and taurine-rich foods should be added to the diet 3–4 times weekly.

Great Pyrenees

Though very different from the Saint Bernard, its nutritional needs are similar.

Husky

Though very different from the Samoyed, its nutritional needs are similar.

Komondor

Of course it's not a puli, but it has similar nutritional requirements.

Kuvasz

His large size, heavy coat, and large body require nutrition similar to that for a Saint Bernard.

Mastiff

This giant short-haired dog makes a wonderful pet, but is not without its problems, which include bone and heart disease, bloat, and ear infections. Food must consist of a high-quality alternative professional food, with alfalfa and torula yeast added daily. L-carnitine- and taurine-rich food can be added two to three times weekly. The alfalfa serves as an antioxidant and supports normal bone growth, and the yeast will add the needed nutrients for the heart. Precautions against bloat are imperative (see p. 73). Puppies less than 2 years of age must be kept thin with steady exercise that does not include jumping.

Newfoundland

Though very different from the Saint Bernard, its nutritional needs are similar.

Portuguese Water Dog

Though this dog has the water-resistant thick coat, oily skin, and hanging ears of a spaniel, it's considered a working dog by the AKC. Its nutritional needs are similar to those of Irish and American spaniels. Some Portuguese water dogs have a genetic disease called Copper Storage Disease and require a low copper diet. (See page 124.)

Rottweiler

With a body like a Mack truck, and the disposition of a guardian angel, this dog requires little maintenance if fed an alternative high-quality food plus vegetable enzymes to keep his muscles, skin, and coat in shape. A good exercise program can develop him into the tight-muscled dog he is known to be. Slow growth is essential for a healthy musculo-skeletal system.

Saint Bernard

This gentle, affectionate giant who can become a fierce guardian must be taken seriously. All precautions against bloat (see p. 73), heart and joint disease must be taken. L-carnitine- and taurine-rich foods must be added to a high-quality alternative professional food, along with alfalfa to help prevent bone disease. Keeping your dog thin until 2 years of age, no Frisbee, and steady exercise will help ensure strong muscles and stable bone development. Daily grooming helps reduce shedding, as will the addition of vegetable enzymes to the diet. Cleaning the ears and eyes daily with goldenseal solution will prevent infections.

Samoyed

This white, fluffy, sturdy, affectionate breed needs an owner who likes to brush and comb. A high-quality protein and fat diet with the addition of vegetable enzymes should keep the coat healthy—if you can get your Samoyed to eat it. They are picky eaters, so leaving food down all day may be the best way to keep them calm and their tummies full. Brewer's yeast and garlic are good treat choices. To stimulate the appetite, try Pet Tinic.

Schnauzer (Standard)

Of the three schnauzers—miniature, standard, and giant (all different breeds)—the standard is the prototype for the others. Its compact, muscled body, flowing feathers on the legs, and notorious skin problems require a high-quality alternative food with the addition of a vegetable enzyme. The giants require bloat prevention (p. 73), slow growth, and L-carnitine- and taurine-rich foods (p. 46). The miniature requires exercise and careful feeding because of the tendency to get fat.

SPORTING GROUP

American Water Spaniel

Don't call him a poodle, whatever you do! While that magnificent curly coat seems to take care of itself, sometimes it gets a little oily down on the skin. Daily antioxidants and an additional vitamin E supplement, combined with a good-quality food should remedy oil problems.

Brittany Spaniel

With their desire to please, excellent sense of smell, and-easy-to-care-for coat, Brittanys are the spaniel of choice for many. Exercise, portion-controlled free-feeding during the day, a hollow bone with peanut butter packed in the middle, and raw vegetables as treats is the way to go for city dogs. Weekend country play can be rewarded with ¼ cooked liver mixed with his food. Don't forget his daily brushing and antioxidant treat.

Chesapeake Bay Retriever

This dog has a thick, short coat with a dense, fine, woolly undercoat, perfect for winter hunting. High-quality food will keep muscles and coat in healthy condition. Antioxidants added to his food or as treats will help extend his life while reducing oiliness in the coat.

Clumber Spaniel

This dog bears little resemblance to a spaniel. His tight, muscular body and long coat with flowing feathers require an alternative food. Exercise is essential to keep him trim.

Cocker Spaniel

One of the most popular breeds, these dogs have health problems. These include hip dysplasia, progressive retinal atrophy, cataracts, and skin disease. While we can't fight genetics, we can try to avoid some of these problems by adding antioxidants to a high-quality protein and fat diet, in the form of oat or wheat grass or alfalfa in their puppy food. Keeping your dog thin will help ensure proper bone and muscle growth. Cleaning the eyes and ears daily should be part of your routine. When you simply don't have the energy to use up his, chamomile tea with warm milk and a biscuit, or Calms Homeopathic Remedy tablets, are useful. Brewer's yeast and garlic treats will supply the B vitamins to help calm, and provide nutrients for skin and coat.

Curly-Coated Retriever

It looks like a spaniel and has similar nutritional requirements. There is no mistaking it for a pointer.

English Setter

Although very different from the Irish setter, this dog has similar nutritional needs.

English Springer Spaniel

Exercise, excitement, and love come to mind when I think of this breed. While weight gain is usually not a problem, boredom is. If their hyperactivity is too much for you, try giving valerian or some Calms Homeopathic Remedy tablets. A hollow bone with peanut butter inside or nondestructible toys are necessary for them. Free-choice feeding of a high-protein and fat food is a good idea; a full stomach should help keep your dog out of mischief while ensuring a beautiful coat. Daily maintenance includes cleaning ears and eyes, and exercise.

Field Spaniel

This long-bodied spaniel has nutritional requirements similar to those of the *Clumber spaniel*.

Flat-Coated Retriever

Although a different breed, its nutritional requirements are similar to those of the Chesapeake Bay retriever.

Golden Retriever

Known for his good disposition, love of water, and thick, water-repellent coat, he's little known for his many problems. Eye, joint, skin, and glandular diseases necessitate the daily addition of antioxidant-packed, bone-supporting alfalfa to his food. Allergies respond to omega-3 fatty acid supplements, brewer's yeast and garlic, and bee pollen. Kelp should be avoided unless you know his thyroid status.

Gordon Setter

His nutritional requirements are similar to those of the other setters. A fatty acid supplement may be required to keep his coat shiny and full.

Irish Setter

This redheaded beauty is a handful if you're not used to an energetic clown. Bloat is a real consideration because they tend to eat too fast and refuse to rest after eating. Besides the usual bloat precautions (see p. 73), wash two or three large rocks and put them into the food dish along with the food. Eating around rocks can slow down any dog, even an Irish setter. Calms Homeopathic Remedy tablets, valerian, and free-feeding should be considered to quell some of their excitement. Exercise is a must, but no jumping before your setter turns 2 years old. Alfalfa added to the high-quality diet he needs for that beautiful red coat will ensure his antioxidant intake. When he becomes too rambunctious, a natural calmer such as valerian or honey will help.

Irish Water Spaniel

The tallest of the spaniels, he has nutritional requirements similar to those of the American and Irish spaniels.

Labrador Retriever

This hunk of muscle and willingness to work requires a high-quality alternative food plus a multivitamin–mineral supplement. He is prone to obesity, so watch those calories. If dandruff or oily skin becomes a problem, supplement with an antioxidant formulation that contains vitamin E.

Pointer

If you saw this dog in point position, you would understand how he got his name. A muscled sportsman, this dog needs daily exercise and a high-quality food to maintain good shape. Food can be left during the day, but it should be portion-controlled. Antioxidants can be given as treats alternately with spirulina, oat or barley grass, or an antioxidant formula. When he becomes too rambunctious, a natural calmer such as valerian or honey will help.

Pointer, German

Though he is different from the pointer, the same nutritional advice applies.

Pointer, German Wire-haired

This pointer requires the same nutrition as the other pointers.

Sussex Spaniel

This short spaniel has the nutritional requirements of the cocker spaniel. As with any floppy-eared dog, the addition of garlic to the diet will help build up resistance to ear infections.

Vizsla

This sleek, well-muscled, floppy-eared dog must have a high-quality alternative food and daily exercise. The exercise helps build muscle and, equally important, will burn up some of that energy this dog seems to have an endless supply of.

Weimaraner

Though he is different from a vizsla, they have similar nutritional requirements. A natural antianxiety supplement is sure to be needed if you keep him in the house or kennel all day. You better leave nondestructible toys for him, because he doesn't like to be confined.

Welsh Springer Spaniel

Though he is different from the cocker spaniel, his nutritional needs are similar.

Wire-haired Pointing Griffon

Muscles, floppy ears, and the wiry, double water-resistant coat give you the hint that it's a spaniel. Its nutritional requirements are similar to those of the Clumber spaniel.

TOY BREEDS

Affenpinscher

A terrier in a compact toy body, this wiry-haired dog does well on any type of diet. His love of play makes him a candidate for portion-controlled free-feeding and for natural antianxiety supplements when required. Go easy on the fattening treats, and be serious about his exercise to keep him in prime condition.

Brussels Griffon

A bundle of personality, this dog needs love first, then a balanced food with a vegetable enzyme to keep his skin and smooth or rough coat healthy. Brewer's yeast and garlic make the perfect treat, adding the protein building blocks necessary for this well-muscled dog.

Cavalier King Charles Spaniel

Who wouldn't fall in love with those big, innocent eyes and that loving personality? Be careful to keep the hanging ears clean, and clean the eyes daily. A high-quality protein and fat food plus a vegetable enzyme will keep that beautiful coat healthy. If your little Cavalier's energy becomes too much to bear, increase exercise, free-feed, and give him chamomile tea with honey, warm milk, and a biscuit.

Chihuahua

Known for their little size, Chihuahuas can have long or short coats. They are wonderful dogs who have no problem being spoiled, but feeding them "people food" makes them very sick. A quality canned dog food, veggies for treats because they tend to get fat, a daily antioxidant treat, and love will keep them healthy.

Chinese Crested

These distinctive dogs, either hairless (long legs, tassel of hair on the head) or powder puff (full, fluffy hair), are known for their sweet personality. Feed them a high-quality high-fat food. This dog loves the outdoors, so sunscreen and daily antioxidants are important. If skin problems occur, a fatty acid supplement and a vegetable enzyme are probably the solution.

English Toy Spaniel

This remarkable bundle of love requires some special care. The hanging ears, potential for oily skin, and all its hair make an alternative professional diet a must. Raw garlic, an immune booster, should be included in all meals. Daily brushing and exercise are necessary, as are antioxidants to protect him from degenerative eye disease.

Italian Greyhound

This sleek, petite, intelligent coursing dog should look anything but frail. Its muscular body and shiny coat require a high-protein, high-fat diet. Oat, wheat, or barley grass, spirulina, or algae added to the food will satisfy his antioxidant requirements. Substitute veggies for biscuits, and give him an occasional knuckle bone to keep him trim and his teeth in good condition.

Japanese Chin

Hair, hair, and more hair with big eyes describes this little dog. Alternative professional food with an enzyme supplement is a must. The enzyme is added for more thorough food digestion and to help digest the hair that gets swallowed when he decides to groom himself. Antioxidants are needed to protect against degenerative eye disease and for overall health.

Maltese

Known for its full coat, this lovely dog requires the same nutritional plan as the Japanese Chin. If he gets a little too rowdy, warm milk (lactose-free) with honey and a biscuit, or an antianxiety supplement can be given.

Miniature Pinscher

No, it isn't a shrunken Doberman! This muscular small version of a Doberman has nutritional needs much like those of the Italian greyhound.

Papillon

A very small spaniel-like dog, this fur ball requires the same nutrition as the Japanese Chin. Exercise and love are the keys to keeping this dog content.

Pekinese

The epitome of royalty, this big-eyed breed has won the hearts of millions and can shed enough to cover them all in excess fur! An alternative professional food with a vegetable enzyme added is a must for good skin and coat. Healthy eyes require daily cleaning and antioxidants included in the diet. Ester C and bee pollen should be given to allergic dogs.

Pomeranian

Looking like a small fox, this witty, alert dog has much the same nutritional needs as the Pekinese. If he gets too vocal for you, try a natural calming remedy such as valerian, wild lettuce, or Calms by Hyland's.

Pug

Their tiny, sweet, pushed-in face, big eyes, and wrinkled skin need a diet of high-quality protein and fat with the addition of antioxidants in a natural food form (grass or algae). If shedding becomes a problem, add a fatty acid supplement.

Shih Tzu

These elegant, big-eyed, long-haired beauties owe their coat to genetics and a high-quality protein and fat diet combined with a vegetable enzyme. Their teeth need raw vegetables, and occasional marrow bones stuffed with peanut butter help to relieve their separation anxiety as will Calms by Hyland's, or chamomile tea with honey and a biscuit. Exercise makes a difference in their musculature. Don't forget to give antioxidants.

Silky Terrier

This toy terrier's beauty comes from his long, silky coat and well-muscled body. An alternative professional food is mandatory, and should be supplemented with vegetable enzymes. Exercise is essential for his mind and body. If time out is needed, try an antianxiety natural supplement.

Yorkshire Terrier

Their silky, flowing coat and loving personalities have lured owners into feeding them people food only, causing all kinds of problems. Dog food with high-quality protein and fat is needed to keep skin, coat, and muscles in good health. The addition of an antioxidant will help ensure many years of joy.

Nonsporting Group

American Eskimo Dog

Whether you have the toy, miniature, or standard, these loyal, playful dogs come with lots and lots of fur! To keep shedding under control and their hair in the soft, full condition it's known for, feeding a high-quality food with the addition of a vegetable enzyme is a must. Brewer's yeast and garlic is your treat of choice for the summer months, and may help improve appetite. Make sure to add antioxidants. Daily exercise is important for their mental and physical health.

Bichon Frise

Often mistaken for poodles, these furry little love balls make wonderful companions. A food without any dyes and with high-quality protein and fat is necessary to maintain a nice coat and, according to breeders, reduce the rusty stains that accumulate under the runny eyes. Bee pollen and antioxidants should be added to their food, the former for its help in fighting allergies.

Boston Terrier

This lively, inquisitive, short-muzzled dog can be a wonderful pet but needs some special care. Eye protection is a must: daily wiping with an eyebright solution and antioxidants added to the food in the form of a grass or algae. Keep them exercised and in good health by feeding veggies rather than biscuits. If their coat gets oily, add a vitamin E supplement along with brewer's yeast and garlic.

Bulldog

This massive, wrinkle-faced dog with broad shoulders and rolling skin is truly a delightful pet, but one that requires nutritional help. The nose, ears, and eyes must be cleaned daily with eyebright solution. Since allergies can be a real problem, quercetin or bee pollen added to a quality protein and fat diet will decrease the allergic response and help keep the immune system strong. Bloat precautions are required (see p. 73). A vegetable enzyme added to the food will help with digestion while sending the necessary nutrients to the skin and coat, another problem area. Fresh garlic should be added to the food and brewer's yeast and garlic should be your treat of choice, along with carrots and celery. Raw vegetables will keep off the fat while cleaning the teeth.

Chinese Shar-Pei

Once the unusual wrinkled dog a yuppie simply couldn't live without, its many problems have decreased its popularity. An alternative professional food, plus a vegetable enzyme and brewer's yeast or spirulina supplement, is your best bet to combat their frequent skin problems. To strengthen their immune system and help fight off joint disease, fresh garlic and alfalfa are a must. If the skin gets too oily, vitamin E supplementation may be helpful.

Chow Chow

With its blue tongue, massive layers of fur, and reputation as a quality guardian and friend, this breed is very popular despite the maintenance involved. One chow owner said that if it wasn't for brewer's yeast and garlic, flea control would be impossible. Feeding a high-quality protein and fat food with the addition of vegetable enzymes will help promote a healthy coat with less shedding.

Dalmatian

For this breed made famous by firemen and Walt Disney, there are a few things you need to know to keep them healthy and both of you happy. If your puppy is too much to handle, a good trainer and a natural calming remedy (such as valerian or milk and honey) is in order. Since they usually are not prone to gain weight until they're older, portion-controlled free-feeding may help keep your puppy calm. A long bone packed with peanut butter may keep him busy, as will other chew-type toys. Many Dalmatians form urate crystals or stones in their kidneys and bladder. Unless your dog has formed these stones, I recommend an alternative high-quality food: medium quantities of protein (low in organ meats) and high in carbohydrates and fats.

Finnish Spitz

Known for his distinctive bark, this husky-looking dog has such a full coat that flea control without brewer's yeast and garlic is frightening. The protein components of the brewer's yeast will help maintain the healthy full coat if you feed this dog a high-quality food.

French Bulldog

Although not a bulldog, this little dog has the same nutritional requirements as a bulldog.

Keeshond

This handsome bundle of fur requires an alternative food to keep his thick, long coat from becoming dull and brittle. I wouldn't think of owning one without brewer's yeast and garlic for summer flea control. It's also the perfect treat to encourage a healthy full coat. Grooming and love are everything.

Lhasa Apso

These dogs have it all—a luxurious coat, big eyes, and dangling, long ears. A high-quality diet with the addition of bee pollen is recommended for skin and coat, and for ear infection control. The addition of vegetable enzymes and antioxidants is an added plus. Daily eye and ear cleaning with eyebright solution must be part of your grooming routine. To help deter kidney disease, B vitamins and omega-3 fatty acids in treat form are recommended.

Poodle

Toy, miniature, or standard, these intelligent, lovable, low-maintenance pets are very popular. Eye protection consists of daily cleaning with eyebright solution and the addition of antioxidants to the food or as a treat. Standard poodles need bone protection with alfalfa added to their food and an owner who keeps them thin. Veggies should be the treat of choice when you're not giving spirulina or brewer's yeast and garlic for additional skin and coat care.

Schipperke

Give this breed antioxidants and feed quality professional food so it can live the long life it's known for and its full, heavy coat can stay healthy. Shedding can be a problem, vegetable enzymes added to the food are helpful.

Tibetan Spaniel

This sweet, gentle, fuzzy dog doesn't require much grooming but does need an alternative high-quality food. Brewer's yeast and garlic treats will reward him as they keep his coat shiny and healthy. If he gets too spirited at times, natural antianxiety remedies will help calm him down. Oily skin demands an antioxidant with vitamin E.

Tibetan Terrier

Looking almost like a sheepdog, this dog has so much hair you can't find the eyes! An alternative high-quality food is a must, with added vegetable enzymes and brewer's yeast and garlic as his favorite treats. Grooming is as necessary as love and exercise.

HERDING GROUP

Australian Cattle Dog

A splendid blend of colors, big ears, and big heart make this maintenance-free dog more popular by the day. He's naturally made to work, so be sure yours has plenty of interactive toys, and lots of exercise morning and evening. If your puppy doesn't want to eat, that's okay, because it's just too busy being involved with life. Free-feed may be the right choice for you. On days when he's just too much to handle, an herbal calmer like valerian, or warm milk with honey, might take the edge off for both of you. Give him antioxidant treats or veggies every time he does something right.

Bearded Collie

This hunk of hair just needs to be cuddled, when not being groomed. High-quality foods plus a vegetable enzyme will help keep the coat from being dull or feeling like cotton. Their natural desire is to play, so an herbal calmer or warm milk and honey may become an early evening ritual. Fleas can be a real problem, so brewer's yeast and garlic should be started as a treat or supplement every spring. Don't forget the antioxidants.

Belgian Malinois

This strong, muscled dog with a short coat can be fed a supermarket food, providing you add a vegetable enzyme and give him nutritious treats. Exercise is essential for his mind and body.

Belgian Sheepdog

All that hair requires an alternative high-quality food that has at least 2–3 cereals in the ingredients. It should be given by portion-controlled free-feeding. Don't be concerned about the coarseness of the hair; that's normal. Brewer's yeast and garlic can be given as healthy fur treats, particularly in the summertime.

Belgian Tervuren

Used once as a herding dog, and now for therapy, this solid dog doesn't require any frills. A supermarket food with a "whole food" (bee pollen) added is perfect.

Border Collie

A very bright dog, it can be a handful for a new owner—not the grooming or the general care, but the training. Use positive reinforcement with healthy treats—no sugar, dyes, or preservatives. The coat thrives on high-quality protein and fat foods. Leaving food down all day should help reduce some of the stress from being alone. When he really gets anxious, calming herbs like valerian can help reduce restlessness.

Bouvier des Flandres

Talk about a big breed full of love, kisses, and hair, and you've described it. All that muscle and hair require a high-quality protein and fat food with the addition of a vegetable enzyme. Take care to prevent bloat (see p. 73), and supplement with alfalfa to prevent bone disease. Brewer's yeast and garlic are helpful for summertime flea, skin, and coat problems.

Briard

This big dog with long hair requires work but is worth it. An alternative professional food, frequent grooming, bloat prevention (see p. 73), and healthy heart supplements (taurine and L-carnitine [p. 46]) are all necessary. Antioxidants should be started at age 2.

Collie

Whether your Lassie is rough- or smooth-haired (the latter has long, flowing hair), it is an exceptional pet that should be fed a high-quality protein and fat food with vegetable enzymes. Antioxidants in the form of oat, wheat, or barley grass or algae should be added to the food for eye and whole body protection.

English Sheepdog

This bundle of fur and love has nutritional needs similar to those of the briard. If your sheepdog gets a little boisterous, try Calms Homeopathic Remedy or add a little oat grass to his food.

German Shepherd

Rin Tin Tin helped to make this strong, alert dog a household breed. Because of its temperamental digestive tract, an alternative professional food is required. Bloat prevention (see p. 73) is a must, as is an antioxidant started at age 2; spirulina or alfalfa is my choice. During shedding season, add vegetable enzymes to the food.

Puli

Long, hanging braids that hide eyes and legs makes this dog unique. The thick, woolly undercoat and outer coat require an alternative food with vegetable enzymes. No puli owner could live through the summer without brewer's yeast and garlic as a supplement or treat. The daily addition of raw garlic to the food will help boost the immune system, and particularly to help avoid eye and ear problems.

Shetland Sheepdog

Looking like a miniature Lassie, these lovable dogs have nutritional needs similar to those of collies.

Welsh Corgi

Whether you have a Cardigan or a Pembroke, chances are that their short legs, long body, and fairly maintenance-free coat made you fall in love. They can become destructive when left alone for long periods of time—after all, they were bred to work. Interactive toys, free-feeding, and an herbal calmer are useful substitutes for work. Both breeds require antioxidant supplementation in the food or as a treat.

CHAPTER SEVEN

Nutritional FAQs

During the many years I've been treating animals with a holistic, natural approach to nutrition, I've been asked for advice in a variety of areas. I've decided to group the most frequently asked questions (FAQs) into one section. I suggest you read through these, especially if you have a question. You just might find the answer.

Q: My puppy, Tiny, is anything but. He is only 4 months old and weighs 50 lbs. Do I continue feeding him puppy food?
A puppy doesn't really have different nutritional needs than a young or middle-aged dog; it just requires more of everything—in the same balance. The best way to provide the additional calories a growing puppy requires is by serving a more concentrated food (with higher calories). Protein is required for growth, either increased protein or better protein. Because a puppy's teeth are smaller than an adult's, a softer dry food may be helpful for a small breed.

If you are feeding a supermarket food, then your puppy probably still requires the puppy food because of its higher protein, fat, and calorie content. If you are feeding him a quality alternative food, the adult version should have everything in it your puppy requires. You will just need to feed more of it than the same brand of puppy food to satisfy his increased nutrient requirements. If he seems to be gaining too much weight on a puppy food (you can't feel the rib cage easily), then adult food is best for him.

Q: *I just bought a 3-month-old German shepherd puppy. His ears won't stand up. The breeder suggested calcium for his ears and bones. Is this correct?*
A: No! All dog food contains more than enough calcium, even some of my least favorite foods. Calcium has nothing to do with your dog's ears standing up straight, despite the myths that have been circulating for years. Ears stand straight because of genetics and proper taping when the dog is young. As far as bone development goes, bones require all types of nutrients to grow strong and healthy. Calcium is one nutrient that simply can't be supplemented. If you absolutely must, add calcium by serving an additional meal of calcium-rich food, such as dairy products.

Q: *My 4-year-old dog, Sally, can't seem to gain weight. The veterinarian said she is fine. She never finishes her food, so I can't fatten her up. What do you suggest?*
A: Sally is probably just a svelte dog that doesn't need to be fattened up. Yet, if you insist, these are my suggestions. Add a vegetable enzyme to her food to increase the amounts of nutrients absorbed into her body. Feed her a high-quality puppy food, 3 or 4 times daily. If she is a small dog, add ⅛ tsp. of corn oil; for a large dog, add ½ tsp. of corn oil to each meal. Walk her up and down the steps, and give her lots of other exercise to get those muscles bulked up.

Q: *My dog has acne on his chin and all around his mouth. Antibiotics clear it up, but only temporarily. Any suggestions?*
A: Check the food dishes you are using. Plastic can cause an allergic reaction; your dog scratches, and creates a secondary infection. I prefer ceramic or steel bowls.

Q: *My dog's eyes tear all the time. It seems that the tears are darker in color lately. What can I do?*
A: If the tearing is due to allergies, give your dog the appropriate supplements for allergy (see p. 49). Make sure the food you're feeding does not contain any dyes or preservatives. Garlic should be added to your dog's food to strengthen his/her immune system. Last, make sure you gently wipe the eyes daily with a piece of cotton moistened with a goldenseal solution.

Q: *Do brewer's yeast and garlic really repel fleas?*
A: One study, perhaps the only one ever done, determined that it does not. However, I owned a boarding kennel and presently live in Florida, the flea capital of the USA. My dogs are all on brewer's yeast and garlic, and only occasionally require a natural flea killer. I believe that the brewer's yeast keeps the skin healthy, so that when the dog scratches and bites at it, there is less damage, and thus, you may think, fewer fleas. The garlic is a natural antibiotic with essential oils; both work with the brewer's yeast to make the skin so healthy that a flea bite or two doesn't affect your dog as much.

Q: My 7-month-old shepherd refuses to eat. I know you're supposed to let them go hungry, but he will go days without eating unless I "doctor up" his food. What do I do?
A: Puppies are notorious for being poor eaters. They are too interested in life to give food a second thought. Unlike us, conditioned to eat at certain times, when they get hungry, they will eat. Your dog has simply been spoiled and is waiting for you to give in and make him an exciting meal. As long as he has no sign of illness and is active, you can win this match. You simply must resist those puppy eyes. Put his food out, and he will eat when he is hungry, provided he isn't ill.

Q: I am feeding my dog Nutramax and Science Diet. Someone told me that I'm wrong. What do you think?
A: Never mix two different brands of food. You can throw off the nutrient balance and harm your dog. If you're feeding a dry food and want to increase its flavor, you can add water, garlic powder, a small amount of canned food made by the same manufacturer, or an all-meat canned dog food that is NOT 100% nutritional.

Q: Why do dogs eat grass? Is this bad for their health?
A: Dogs will search out roughage if not enough is being provided by the diet. You may want to grow a pot of barley grass or wheat grass for him to nibble on when he wants. Another alternative is to add wheat bran or oat bran to his food. You may want to try my favorite combination of half debittered brewer's yeast and half bran. Small dogs can start with ⅛ tsp. per meal, and large dogs can start with ½ tsp. You can increase the amount slowly every week, but keep in mind that increased fiber can also mean increased stool frequency and quantity.

Q: I am having difficulty housebreaking my dog. He urinates in his crate, so I have not been leaving him water during the day. I'm not sure if that is harmful to him. Any suggestions?
A: Get him examined by his veterinarian to make sure he doesn't have a urinary tract infection. Don't *ever* limit water—unless instructed to do so by your veterinarian. You can help reduce the amount of water he drinks by buying a dry food with a lower salt (sodium) content. Generally speaking, supermarket foods have higher salt levels than quality alternative foods. Dry food is preferable to canned because there is generally 10% water in dry food, while it can be as high at 78% in canned food.

Q: How can I eliminate worms naturally?
A: I deliberately did not include worms in the problem/solution list because that is something that should be left to your family veterinarian. While there are herbs that kill worms in dogs, a natural deworming program is complicated. To be done correctly, it must include fasting and liver

detoxification. Today's wormers are so safe that I feel it's unreasonable to use anything else.

Q: *How can I increase my dog's appetite?*
A: There is no easy answer, because a poor appetite can be due to many things. A veterinarian visit is necessary to rule out disease. Dogs with liver, kidney, or other debilitating problems will generally lose their appetites. B vitamins and zinc are always helpful supplements. Puppies tend to be picky eaters, so don't be alarmed if they don't empty the bowl the minute you set it down. You can increase the flavor and appeal of the food by adding garlic powder, liver powder, or a small amount of chicken fat.

Q: *One of my two dogs has cataracts, but the other one hasn't developed them yet. What can be done naturally to decrease the risk of cataracts in my other dog?*
A: Cataracts can be caused by anything that will damage the lens of the eye, which includes poor nutrition, injury, oxidative stress (free radicals), and diseases that affect blood flow to the eye. Your primary defense should include a high-quality dog food and the addition of antioxidants.

Q: *My dog is 4 years old and has horrible breath. It can't be his teeth, because he eats only dry food and nibbles on biscuits during the day. What do you think?*
A: Offensive breath is usually caused by stomach and/or intestinal problems, or teeth and gums that need a good cleaning. To rule out intestinal disease, a visit to the family veterinarian is useful. Bring a stool sample that can can be checked for worms. Your dog should be on a high-quality food fed at least twice daily, with vegetable enzymes added. Chopped peppermint or parsley can be added to the food to sweeten the breath. B vitamins or brewer's yeast should be used as a supplement. Contrary to old-fashioned belief that dry food is healthier for teeth and gums than canned food, dry food may not clean teeth and gums, especially in dogs that inhale rather than chew their food. If the dry food you are serving is small, search for one with larger pieces, preferably by the same manufacturer. Many dogs have remained tartar-free when fed Hills Prescription T/d, a dry food that is formulated to have additional teeth-cleaning qualities. Good oral hygiene requires chew toys and treats, some of which have enzymes in them that discourage bacterial growth. Veterinarian-only chew rawhide with enzymes is available, providing your dog can be given rawhide. Daily teeth brushing and a yearly cleaning by your family veterinarian is very helpful.

Q: *My dog bites his foot all day long, causing it to become raw, infected, and swollen. I've tried everything. What can I do?*
A: Foot biting can result from separation or just plain anxiety, or become a habit after the dog is bitten by a flea or mosquito. Sometimes excessive biting and licking start off as a means of getting attention; every time the dog

bites, the owner chastises the dog, giving it attention—positive or negative, it doesn't matter. To alleviate the need for attention, spend time with your dog at least twice daily. When he does lick, ignore it. At the same time, treat him naturally for anxiety (p. 51). Omega-3 fatty acids will help eliminate some of that itching. Ask your veterinarian for an antihistamine at the proper dosage, to aid in itch reduction. Studies show that when omega-3 fatty acids are combined with an antihistamine, results can be remarkable. Since every dog differs in its antihistamine response, you may need to ask your veterinarian for several. If all else fails, your dog may be classified as obsessive-compulsive and require a mood elevator, such as Elavil, prescribed by your veterinarian.

Q: I breed tiny Yorkshire terriers and Chihuahuas. Why can't I feed them baby food while they're weaning?
A: Baby food is made for human babies, not for dogs. It does not have nearly enough nutritional components for your dogs to grow up healthy. Most people feed meat baby food, and then a vegetable and a fruit. Chances are that you're feeding only the meat baby food, which is almost devoid of calcium and has too much phosphorus. All-meat baby food causes all-meat syndrome which is essentially calcium deficiency.

Q: Why is chocolate poisonous to dogs?
A: Chocolate contains a substance called theobromine, which is toxic in dogs if it is eaten in large quantities. Symptoms include vomiting, diarrhea, panting, and muscle tremors, within 4–5 hours after eating the chocolate. Since we are not sure about the amount that causes irreversible damage, your best bet is to avoid all chocolate—and any cocoa or chocolate-flavored treat.

Q: Can I give my dog my multivitamin product? He weighs almost 120 pounds.
A: While it probably would not hurt to do so, dogs need a different balance of nutrients than we do. If you are going to support his health with supplements, why not provide him with one that is formulated for dogs?

Q: When I supplement my dogs with garlic, I use garlic powder. Is that okay?
A: It depends upon why you are using the garlic. If you want to improve the taste of your dog's food, garlic powder (without the salt) is perfect. If you are giving garlic as a nutrient—to strengthen his immune system and resistance to insects, and to enhance his skin and coat—then you need to use fresh garlic. You can cut a clove into small pieces and give a small dog ¼ of an average-sized clove, a medium dog ½, and a large dog the entire clove. As with anything you add to your dog's food, start with a small amount and gradually work up to the proper amount. If you don't want the odor of garlic on your hands, crushed or chopped garlic is available in the supermarket.

Q: I can't get my dog off the semimoist food. I know it's not good for him, but he'd rather starve than eat anything else. Help!

A: While I am not a proponent of starving a dog into submission, I do need you to be strong with him. Feed him PRIOR to the preparation and eating of your meal, so he doesn't smell something better than the new food you want him to try. It may be easier to switch from semimoist to canned rather than dry. That's okay, because once he is on canned, you can sneak dry food in little by little, until he is eating all dry food or mostly dry food. Place the canned food in his dish and walk away. Leave him alone for 5–15 minutes. If he has not touched it, pick it up. No treats, no table scraps. But love is certainly warranted. The next meal should be done the same way. Small breeds can easily go 24 hours without eating, while medium and large breeds can go 2–3 days. Some experts will have you withhold food for a week, small or large dog. If your dog simply won't switch foods, then put the semimoist food into the dish but cut it into small pieces. Add a small amount of canned food and mix, coating the semimoist food. Refrigerate the rest of the canned food and repeat for the next meal, gradually adding more canned food and less semimoist. Be sure to warm the canned food before you give it to him, because cold food just doesn't taste good.

Q: I am a vegetarian, and don't even wear leather. I refuse to give my dog meat, so I am cooking for him. I prepare grains, nuts, soy, and dairy, just as I do for myself. Then, just in case, I give him a multivitamin supplement. Is that okay?

A: Absolutely not. Dogs need meat and the fat that goes along with it, and they need balanced nutrition. I am willing to bet that your meals are not balanced, at least not for a dog. If you insist on him being a veg head, there are a few vegetarian foods that are 100% nutritional. Keep in mind, however, that those foods are NOT optimum and your dog probably will not reach his full genetic potential and probably will have a dull, dry coat.

Q: My dog doesn't have any teeth but insists on eating dry food. Is that okay?

A: Chances are that your dog lost his teeth a few at a time, allowing his gums to get hard enough for him to "gum" his dry food. As long as he is chewing, even though it's with his gums, it's okay. If he is swallowing the food whole, then you need to change him to a canned food.

Q: My dog eats his stools. What can I do about that?

A: Stool eating can be attributed to behavior learned when he was a puppy. Every litter has a "cleanup" puppy who is required to keep the den clean. If your puppy was the one, then he's still doing his job. Try to make the stools distasteful to him by adding Forbid (veterinarian only) or Deter (in the pet shop) to his food. Some people have success adding canned spinach. Stool eating can also be due to lack of food and or nutrients. If you are feeding a supermarket food, you better beef it up now. If you are feeding an alternative food, make sure it is professional. If your dog is not fat, you may want to increase the quantity of food. Vitamin supplementation is also a must. Stool eating is also a means of getting attention, good or bad. When you see your dog eating his or another dog's stool, don't say or do anything. Try to get to the stools before your dog does, and add the hottest Tabasco or hot sauce you can find, so he rejects them on his own.

Vitamins and Minerals

VITAMINS

This appendix on vitamins and minerals reflects the newest information regarding their use in treating disease and also explains their fundamental disease-prevention roles within the body. To supplement or not to supplement, to use synthetic or natural forms, how often and how much. Every vitamin and mineral is explained briefly, including how it benefits your dog, how much should be given to a healthy dog as a preventive, and the dosages for treatment of specific diseases. Often I will discuss the requirements of certain nutrients as per the American Association of Feed Control Officials (AAFCO). They are responsible for creating minimum and maximum requirements of nutrients for dogs and cats.

Vitamin A

Vitamin A is a fat-soluble vitamin that requires sufficient fats and minerals in order for proper absorption to take place. There are two forms of this vitamin: preformed vitamin A (called retinol), found only in meats, and provitamin A (called beta-carotene), found primarily in plants. Beta-carotene is an antioxidant and does not have to be converted to vitamin A for its antioxidant effect. Because it is a fat-soluble vitamin, it can be stored in the dog's body. An oversupply (for instance, feeding liver or cod liver oil daily) can cause problems. Symptoms include diarrhea, painful neck movements, skeletal problems, and liver disease.

Benefits

• Increases immunity and aids in the prevention of urinary tract and respiratory infections

• Promotes bone and body growth, fertility, good skin and coat, and healthy bones

• Helps pituitary gland function

• Improves vision, hearing, and digestion

• As an antioxidant, provides protection against toxins

Amount

All commercially prepared dog food contains at least the AAFCO minimum requirements; some contain 10 times that much. Vitamin A is not as toxic as once thought. Supplement with 10,000 IU (medium-sized dog, approx. 40 lbs.) daily for 5 days, then stop for 2 days. It works best in conjunction with zinc.

Sources

Liver, kidney, egg yolk, asparagus, broccoli, cantaloupe, carrots, dandelions, parsley, peaches, sweet potatoes, spinach, spirulina, pumpkin, yellow squash, barley grass, wheat grass, alfalfa.

Deficiency Symptoms

Loss of appetite, muscle weakness, weight loss, dull or brittle coat, scaly, hairless patches on skin, conjunctivitis, gum disease, retinal degeneration, intolerance of light, resistance to petting, seizures, and impaired fertility.

Advice

Vitamin A is generally supplemented for a specific health problem, or for poor skin and coat. Many breeders use cod liver oil because it provides the fat for the skin and coat, as well as the vitamin A. The problem with cod liver oil is the potential for vitamin D and vitamin A overdosage, especially if combined with a food whose major ingredients include liver or by-products. Beta-carotene is better known for its antioxidant effects than vitamin A. Both work best as antioxidants when combined with other antioxidants and their support nutrients. To be absolutely sure the balance of antioxidants is correct, you can seldom go wrong with nature, home-grown or store-bought. The daily addition of wheat sprouts, alfalfa, or any of the vegetables mentioned above will cover your dog's daily preventive antioxidant requirement.

B1 (Thiamine)

B1 is a water-soluble member of the B complex; any excess is excreted instead of being stored in the dog's body. It must be replaced daily. Cooking, extended storage, sulfa drugs, air, and water can destroy its potency. It is more effective when taken with other B vitamins, particularly B2 (riboflavin) and B6 (pyridoxine) than alone.

Benefits
- Stimulates the appetite

- Keeps the nervous system, muscles, and heart functioning normally

- Improves attitude, behavior, and intelligence

- Is necessary for healthy carbohydrate metabolism

Amount
Though all commercial dog foods contain at least the minimum AAFCO requirements for B1 (after cooking), supplementing 50–100 mg (for an average-sized dog, 40 lbs.) daily is safe and can be helpful. Thiamine works best if combined with other B vitamins. Sulfa drugs, antibiotics, and high-carbohydrate diets can increase the need for it.

Sources
Egg yolks, organ meats (liver, kidney, heart), pork, chicken, brewer's yeast, torula yeast, bee pollen, soybeans, wheat germ, whole grains, beans, broccoli, nuts, and prunes.

Deficiency Symptoms
Loss of appetite (anorexia), loss of muscle coordination, vomiting, weight loss, fatigue, irritability, and nervousness. Dogs with kidney disease usually need supplementation of all B vitamins, including B1.

Advice
If you want to add thiamine to your dog's diet to help its coat and general well-being, then brewer's or torula yeast is what you want. Loaded with all the B family, plus support nutrients, it is available in chewable wafer, liquid, or powder form. Add garlic to it, and you can take the bite out of fleas. If you're not a yeast fan, add any of the above-mentioned sources to your dog's food (no more than 15%, please). Wheat germ, bee pollen, and egg yolks will do wonders for your dog's coat.

There are instances in which thiamin is needed to treat disease. It should be combined with the other B team members (unless otherwise prescribed by your veterinarian). There are various B complex formulas available that include the B vitamins and support nutrients. Use B1 for stressful conditions such as surgery, traveling, or boarding. It's essential for diabetic dogs, those with kidney disease, or those with any chronic debilitating disease.

B2 (Riboflavin)

This is another member of the water-soluble family of the B complex that cannot be stored in your dog's body and needs to be replaced regularly. Riboflavin is easily absorbed and easily excreted. Depending on your dog's requirements, excretion may be accompanied by protein loss. It is not destroyed by heat or oxidation, but does dissolve in cooking liquids and is destroyed by light.

Benefits

- Very important in the prevention of eye problems, including cataracts

- Aids in the metabolism of all your dog's other nutrients (proteins, fats, and carbohydrates)

- Prevents dry, cracking skin

- Essential during pregnancy

- Helpful for nervous dogs because of its importance in tryptophan metabolism

- Helps protect the intestinal tract when combined with vitamin A or beta-carotene

- Important component for a healthy immune system

Recommended Amount

As with the other B vitamins, all commercial pet food manufacturers include at least the minimum AAFCO requirements. Supplement 50–100 mg. daily for the average-sized dog. Remember, it works best combined with the other B team members.

Sources

Cheese, fish, eggs, chicken, yogurt, cottage cheese, asparagus, avocados, broccoli, nuts, brewer's yeast, torula yeast, bee pollen.

Deficiency Symptoms

Loss of appetite, weight loss, cataracts, hair loss, dry, crusty skin, anemia.

Advice

If your dog is under stress (moving, traveling, boarding) or has any type of chronic illness, you want this vitamin and the other B members included in the daily supplementation. Many breeders supply their pregnant dogs and puppies with all the B2 they need by giving a daily additional meal of cottage cheese. Cottage cheese offers a natural supply of calcium without upsetting the delicate calcium mechanism of the mom or her pups. Strenuous exercise programs should be accompanied by B2 (and the other B vitamins) supplementation. Brewer's or torula yeast is an easy way to provide it. Since additional B2 can interfere with anticancer drugs, talk to your veterinarian before using it if your dog is undergoing cancer therapy.

B3 (Niacin, Niacinamide, Nicotinic Acid)

Another water-soluble member of the B vitamin team, it must be replaced daily. It is easily destroyed by cooking, food processing, sulfa drugs, and water. Niacin is essential for the formation of tryptophan, and it is important for hormones: sex hormones, cortisol, and thyroxin (produced by the thyroid gland). B3 also aids in the functioning of the nervous system and plays an important role in circulation.

Benefits

- Helps increase energy levels

- Useful for behavior problems because it helps to promote a healthy nervous system

- Aids in eliminating mouth sores and bad breath

Recommended Amount

This B vitamin is included as per the AAFCO minimum requirements, or more, in every dog food. Even though it is considered a water-soluble vitamin, and therefore "okay in high doses," it can have adverse effects. It is usually safe in the amounts found in brewer's and torula yeast, but supplementation should not exceed 100 mg daily. Use caution when supplementing dogs with glaucoma, liver disease, and diabetes, and pregnant dogs. Because it can dilate the blood vessels, too much can cause itching and discomfort to your dog. It should NOT be supplemented in dalmatians because of the possibility of increased uric acid production.

Sources

Beef, broccoli, cheese, fish, dairy products, pork, potatoes, tomatoes, organ meats, brewer's or torula yeast.

Deficiency Symptoms

Diarrhea, mouth ulcers, loss of appetite, and chronic respiratory problems.

Advice

As useful as this vitamin is, it has its limitations because of the way the body metabolizes it. I prefer that you supplement with a food from the above list rather than with a store-bought niacin supplement, unless it's a B complex formulation. Time-release niacin must be avoided.

B5 (Pantothenic Acid, Calcium Pantothenate, and Panthenol)

Another member of the B vitamin team, it's important in overall immune support. B5 is very important for the proper function of the adrenals and other glands, and is an essential antistress vitamin. It is easily destroyed by canning, heat, food processing and sulfa drugs. Used as a memory vitamin, it is useful (in a B combination) for training, and important for the normal functioning of the intestinal tract.

Benefits

- Helps to prevent and fight infection by building antibodies
- Helps raise a dog's stress threshold
- Helps to relieve allergies
- Helps in healing of wounds
- Useful in treating sadness and anxiety

Recommended Amount

Like all the other B vitamins, dog food manufacturers include at least the AAFCO minimum requirement in foods and are certain to add the additional amount needed because some is destroyed by heat during production. An average dog (40 lbs.) can be supplemented with 50–100 mg. daily, preferably in combination with the other B vitamins.

Sources

Liver, kidney, egg yolk, wheat germ or wheat bran, chicken, green vegetables, saltwater fish, brewer's yeast and bee pollen.

Deficiency Symptoms

Weight loss, general laziness, fatty liver disease, irritability, and increased susceptibility to allergies.

Advice

Vitamins B5, B6, and B9 are the SWAT team protectors of your dog's immune system. These three vitamins should be supplemented in your dog's diet, no matter what food you are feeding. While supplementation is effective in a multiple B–C vitamin complex, it can also be done by feeding your dog dried liver treats, soft-boiled eggs, or cooked liver 3–4 times weekly (too much liver can cause diarrhea). This is a must for any upcoming stressful event (spaying, neutering, travel, competition, etc.). Allergic dogs should be supplemented with this and the other B vitamins. Brewer's yeast is NOT the supplement of choice, however, for an allergic dog, since it can be a highly reactive, allergic source of B vitamins!

B6 (Pyridoxine)

This is the superstar of the water-soluble B vitamins, though it is excreted with ease and needs daily replenishment. It is essential for the proper digestion of protein and fat, as well as for effective absorption of vitamin B12 (cobalamin) and other nutrients. An absolute must for the production of healthy red blood cells and antibodies, it is easily destroyed by long storage, food processing techniques, canning, cooking, and water.

Benefits
- Aids in the assimilation of protein and fat
- Fortifies the immune system (especially when accompanied by pantothenic and folic acids)
- Improves behavior by preventing many nervous disorders
- Helps to alleviate skin problems
- Enables proper utilization of essential minerals
- Useful in treating sadness and anxiety
- Essential for a healthy nervous system

Recommended Amount
As with all major vitamins, all dog food manufacturers include at least the minimum AAFCO requirements in their food. Supplementation of an average dog (40 lbs.) should be about 50–100 mg., combined with the other B team members.

Sources
Brewer's yeast, torula yeast, wheat bran, wheat germ, organ meats (kidney, liver, heart), egg yolk, cantaloupe, bee pollen, peas and avocado.

Deficiency Symptoms
Skin and coat problems (thin, brittle dry coat, head hanging like an old dog, short whiskers, eyes not bright and alert), nervousness, neurological problems (seizures, nervous tics), weight loss, unthrifty appearance, anemia, conjunctivitis.

Advice

This very important vitamin is too vital to take for granted; that's why every dog, especially puppies and seniors, should be supplemented with a multiple B vitamin or one of the natural whole foods mentioned above. If your dog is having behavior problems, then B6 and its other team members should be started today!

Stress can really deplete B vitamins, especially this one. Stress causes can vary from your dog being left alone all day to being boarded. It's always best to start your dog on a B complex, or a natural substance containing it, at least a week before the expected stress begins.

If your dog has any type of neurological problems (or has recently undergone surgery), this vitamin, along with the other B vitamins, should be given. It's such an important support nutrient that it is used to help many other conditions, including arthritis, hot spots, diabetes, and (always) kidney disease.

B9 (Folic Acid, Folacin, Vitamin M)

A water-soluble member of the B complex, B9 is essential to the healthy development and maintenance of your dog's body—as a puppy, adult, and senior. It is one of the stress fighters, builds antibodies, and is required for the utilization of proteins. It's necessary to make red blood cells, and is thus a treatment for anemia. It can be destroyed by heat, water, sunlight, and sulfa drugs.

Benefits

• Helps develop a powerful immune system

• Considered a brain food, a must for training (in conjunction with the other B team members)

• Supplementation is essential during pregnancy (one of the few times it can be taken without its B family members)

• Stimulates the appetite

• Energizes

Recommended Amount

All pet food manufacturers add the AAFCO minimum required amounts, and some add a little more. Unlike the other B vitamins, a little goes a long way, so 400–800 mcg. is enough for a medium-sized dog unless your veterinarian recommends more.

Sources

Brewer's yeast, torula yeast, organ meats (liver, kidney, heart), egg yolk, cantaloupe, dark green leafy vegetables.

Deficiency Symptoms

Anemia, weakness, impaired growth, diarrhea, lack of appetite.

Advice

A good B complex supplement will give your dog a sufficient amount of folic acid, which is required in only minute amounts. If your dog is ill or fighting off a disease, more folic acid is required. If you're not sure that folic acid is what your dog needs, just add brewer's yeast or bee pollen; either one has all the B vitamins.

Pregnant dogs and lactating ones should be on a B complex supplement or brewer's yeast or Pet Tinic (my favorite tonic, sold only through veterinarians).

If your dog is anemic, chances are your veterinarian already has him on a folic acid supplement.

Vitamin B12 (Cobalamin)

B12, a water-soluble member of the B complex, is quite effective in small doses. It is the only vitamin that also contains essential mineral components. On commercial food labels, it is often listed as the additive cobalamin concentrate or cyanocobalamin. Its absorption can be impaired by a poorly functioning thyroid or malabsorption syndrome. It is found only in animal sources, not plants or vegetables.

Benefits

- Improves the immune system and prevents anemia

- Aids in effective metabolization of protein, fat, and carbohydrates

- Promotes a healthy nervous system

- Promotes growth and increases appetite in puppies and young adults

- A supplement must if your dog is a vegetarian

Recommended Amount

Pet food manufacturers include enough B12 to satisfy the AAFCO minimum requirements and to maintain balance between all the other vitamins. Supplementation should not exceed 100 mcg. for a medium-sized dog, unless otherwise specified by the family veterinarian.

Sources

Organ meats (liver, kidney and heart), fish, dairy products, beef, pork.

Deficiency Symptoms

Gastrointestinal problems including constipation, anemia, impaired growth, susceptibility to infection, abnormal gait.

Advice

If your dog is being fed a quality dog food, and if you are adding organ meat at least 3 times weekly, chances are your dog is not going to have a B12 deficiency. Dogs with pancreatic insufficiency (malabsorption) require additional B12, regardless of the food being fed. Often the best way to give B12 to dogs who lack pancreatic enzymes (necessary to absorb nutrients, especially B12) is by injection.

Since B12 is not normally found in vegetables or cereal grains, a dog whose owner feeds only a vegetarian diet without adequate supplementation is jeopardizing the health of the dog. It is very difficult, if not impossible, to know exactly how much B12 (or any nutrient, for that matter) should be added to match the nutrients in a particular diet.

Dogs evolved as carnivores, and should remain so, eating by-products that include kidney and liver.

Biotin (Vitamin H, Coenzyme R)

This water-soluble member of the B complex is required in small amounts and aids in synthesis of vitamin C. This is necessary for effective metabolism of protein, fat, and carbohydrates. Biotin works synergistically with riboflavin, niacin, pyridoxine, and vitamin A in keeping a dog's skin and coat healthy. Food-processing techniques, water, sulfa drugs, and raw egg whites can destroy its effectiveness. It is produced in the intestines by the breakdown of foods and bacterial fermentation.

Benefits

- Essential for a healthy skin and coat
- Aids in maintaining proper thyroid and adrenal gland function
- Promotes a healthy nervous system
- Assists in optimal metabolization of food

Recommended Amount

As with all the vitamins, dog food manufacturers have added the AAFCO minimum requirements to the food. If you're supplementing, it takes only a little bit: 300–600 mcg. for the average 40-lb. dog.

Sources

Brewer's yeast, torula yeast, egg yolk, beef, liver, kidney, milk, chicken.

Deficiency Symptoms

Scaly skin, dull coat, runny eyes, loss of appetite, weight loss, bloody diarrhea.

Advice

This is a really important vitamin for puppies as well as adults, and especially for seniors. Raw eggs are a no-no because the raw egg white will bind the biotin, making it unavailable to the body. Make sure that any fats you give your dog are fresh, because rancid fats will make the biotin unavailable. Most fatty acid supplements or those for skin and coat will include biotin. If your dog is on sulfa medication or antibiotics, chances are its biotin is being depleted and you need to supplement it. If your dog doesn't have an intolerance to dairy products, the daily addition of yogurt (which contains the natural acidophilus culture) will help the intestines produce biotin.

Choline and Inositol

These water-soluble members of the B complex work together in metabolizing fats. They form lecithin and are essential for the liver.

Benefits

- Helps the liver eliminate poisons and drugs from the body
- Enhances nerve impulse transmission and improves memory
- Modifies excitability and produces a calming effect

Recommended Amount

500–1000 mcg. is adequate supplementation of choline or inositol for the average 40-lb. dog.

Sources

Egg yolk (no raw egg whites), organ meats, wheat germ, brewer's yeast, green leafy vegetables, and cantaloupe.

Deficiency Symptoms

Fat accumulation in the liver, rough, scaly skin, nervousness, gastric ulcers, constipation.

Advice

Dog food manufacturers add these vitamins to their food. If your dog is particularly nervous, or you are about to start his training sessions, then supplement by all means. Don't supplement with choline if your dog has liver disease or has a history of seizures.

Vitamin C (Ascorbic Acid, Cevitamic Acid)

This is a water-soluble vitamin that dogs synthesize in sufficient amounts in their liver (but not enough during stressful situations). Excreted in the urine, it is used up rapidly during growth, stress, or illness, especially if there is an injury to bones. Cooking, heat, light, water, and exposure to air can easily destroy it. It is absolutely essential in forming collagen, the primary constituent for connective tissue, bone, and cartilage. It's also necessary for growth and repair of your dog's teeth, gums, and other tissues, and for helping to absorb iron. On pet food or supplement labels, it appears as the additive ascorbic acid or sodium ascorbate or Ester C.

Benefits
• Improves the immune system and aids in preventing or lessening many types of viral and bacterial infections

• Helps control allergies

• Provides protection from toxins—a major antioxidant

• Helps build strong teeth, gums, and bones, and retards destruction of them as the dog ages

• Aids in preventing urinary tract infections

• Helps counteract side effects of steroids that interfere with collagen formation

• Can relieve joint paint; used to treat arthritis, panosteitis, and osteochondrosis (OCD)

• Beneficial in treating cancer, kidney disease, heart disease

• Speeds up healing after surgery

• The antistress vitamin

Recommended Amount
Because dogs manufacture their own vitamin C, the AAFCO does not consider it necessary. Supplementation depends on the reason: a sudden acute illness, a chronic illness, to reduce stress, or as an antioxidant.

To reduce stress:

50–75 mg. for a small dog (under 15 lbs)

75–100 mg. for a medium dog (approx. 40 lbs)

200–350 mg. for a large dog

350–750 mg. for a giant dog

For acute illness or stress such as surgery, parvo virus, strains or sprains, and wounds:

75–100 mg. for a small dog (under 15 lbs)

200–300 mg. for a medium dog (approx. 40 lbs)

500–1,500 mg. for a large dog

1000–2,500 mg. for a giant dog

For chronic illness, such as allergies, tooth and gum disease, arthritis, diabetes:

50–75 mg. for a small dog

100–200 mg. for a medium dog

250–500 mg. for a large dog

750–1,000 for a giant dog

For antioxidant protection:

25–50 mg. for a small dog

50–75 mg. for a medium dog

100–250 mg. for a large dog

250–500 mg. for a giant dog

Sources

Tomato juice, fruits, vegetables (broccoli, avocados, brussels sprouts, green peas, turnip greens, string beans), liver, bee pollen, wheat grass, barley grass, oat grass.

Deficiency Symptoms

Inflammation of the gums (gingivitis), joint and muscle pain, fatigue, brittle bones, easy bruising, chronic illnesses.

Advice

Vitamin C affects your dog's overall health and well-being. Studies have shown that it strengthens the immune system and can be effective in blocking the destruction caused by viral and bacterial invasion while keeping the support systems of the body healthy. While it's claimed that dogs make enough vitamin C to meet their needs, supplementation is necessary. The trick in vitamin C supplementation is to begin it prior to full-blown symptoms, in high, frequent doses. Oversupplementation or the wrong type of vitamin C can irritate the digestive system, causing your dog to vomit or have diarrhea. The following rules must be remembered when supplementing with vitamin C:

1. Always start with a small dose, increasing it daily until you are giving the required amount. You may find that your dog does well at a certain dosage, but adding to that upsets his or her stomach. If that is the case, accept it, and give only what your dog can tolerate. Many natural veterinarians will give dogs intravenous injections of vitamin C, so that large amounts can be given without side effects. The recommended supplementation amounts given above for acute disease are for ORAL supplementation.

2. Although ascorbic acid is the same for humans as it is for dogs, the acidic form has a bitter taste that your dog may not like. It is usually disguised for humans in a fruit base (cherry, orange, etc.), but many dogs don't like citrus. Manufacturers know that the dog has special tastes, and usually combine it with flavoring that will be acceptable to the dog or use a type of vitamins C that is not acidic, sodium ascorbate.

3. Ester C is a new and special type of vitamin C that is buffered by binding it to amino acids. It doesn't have an acidic taste and is utilized more efficiently than ascorbic acid. As a matter of fact, 500 mg. of Ester C is just about equivalent to 1,000 mg. of ascorbic acid, so you use less.

4. If your dog has a history of urinary tract disease (bladder or kidney), ask your vet about vitamin C supplementation. There has always been concern about the formation of kidney or bladder stones with high or prolonged vitamin C supplementation.

5. If you're supplementing with vitamin C, chances are you need to include other antioxidants, support nutrients, or whole food supplements such as bee pollen, wheat grass, or algae.

6. Avoid supplementing vitamin C in puppies under 6 months unless you are doing so for panosteitis or per your veterinarian. Though breeders will tell you that it doesn't affect bone growth, it does—and can interfere with calcium usage.

Vitamin D

Vitamin D is often called "the sunshine vitamin." Ultraviolet rays acting on the dog's skin oils produce the vitamin, which is then absorbed into the body. When obtained through food (essentially fish oils and liver), it is absorbed with fats through the intestinal walls. Vitamin D can be stored in the body and does not require daily replenishment. (An oversupply can cause hypervitaminosis D; an uneven distribution of calcium in the bones and even in organs such as heart, kidney, and lungs; abnormal teeth; vomiting; pain; and stiffness.) On food labels, it is often listed as the additive calciferol, ergocalciferol, or cholecalciferol.

Benefits
- Promotes strong bones and teeth
- Prevents osteoporosis and rickets
- Stimulates the immune system

Recommended Amount
The AAFCO requirement for adult dogs is 11 IU per kg. of body weight. Unless it is included in a supplement, don't give it to your dog without your veterinarian's approval.

Sources
Sunlight, egg yolk (no uncooked eggs), fish oils, liver and fish.

Deficiency Symptoms
Rickets in the young and osteomalacia in adults. The latter is a bone deformity in which the jaw becomes movable, thus called "rubber jaw," which leads to tooth loss.

Advice
This is one vitamin I don't want you to supplement unless your veterinarian tells you otherwise. Realizing that many dogs just don't get enough sunlight, all pet food manufacturers have added vitamin D to their food, some of them adding 10 times more than required. Vitamin D toxicity can be very insidious and dangerous. Don't worry about rickets in your puppy, because it has become a very rare disease that is usually due to a hormone imbalance in your dog. If you feel that your dog must have additional vitamin D, then feed it liver 3 times weekly. (Excess liver causes diarrhea in many dogs.) Supplementation with cod liver oil, done in the old days, is also a no-no. Cod liver oil contains vitamins D and A, both of which are found in very high quantities in most dog foods.

Vitamin E

This is a fat-soluble vitamin that, unlike some others (A, D, and K) is stored only for a relatively short time in the body, and is extremely safe. It is an important antioxidant (currently found in natural foods and treats). It prevents oxidation of fat compounds, vitamin A, selenium, some vitamin C, and other nutrients. Vitamin E can be destroyed by food processing, extremes in temperature, iron, chlorine, and mineral oil. It often appears on food labels as the additive alpha-tocopherol acetate, alpha-tocopherol concentrate, or alpha-tocopherol acid succinate. Vitamin E can be in a natural or synthetic form.

Benefits

- Strengthens the immune system

- Provides protection against environmental pollutants and toxins

- Retards cellular aging, boosts endurance, and improves the functioning of all organs

- Helps cure skin problems

- Oxygenates the blood and keeps the circulatory system healthy

- Essential for a healthy reproductive system

- Essential for healthy eyes

Recommended Amount

The required amount depends on the diet: the more fat in the diet, the more vitamin E is necessary. The minimum AAFCO requirement is 1.1 mg per kilo of body weight. For average antioxidant supplementation, the following are recommended:

Small dogs, 50–100 IU every other day

Medium dogs, 125–250 IU every other day

Large dogs, 250–400 IU every other day

Giant dogs, 400–600 IU every other day

Sources

Liver, wheat germ, green leafy vegetables (broccoli, spinach), egg yolk, cold-pressed vegetable oils, sweet potatoes, oatmeal.

Deficiency Symptoms

Poor skin and coat, fatigue, reproductive problems, eye problems, chronic diseases.

Advice

Truly a remarkable vitamin antioxidant, vitamin E is not as toxic as was previously thought. Care must be taken NOT to oversupplement with this or any other antioxidant, because at certain levels (not yet identified), the antioxidant effects become the opposite—and you are actually doing harm rather than good! Greasy dogs with dandruff generally need vitamin E supplementation (at above recommended dosages). Since vitamin E works best when it is combined with selenium, vitamin C, and beta-carotene, look for these in the vitamin E supplement you select. Barley, wheat, or oat grass, spirulina, and wheat germ are balanced the way nature thinks best and contain the vitamin E support nutrients required. But while the natural form of vitamin E is probably more useful to the body than the synthetic form, the natural form is very expensive and not as readily available as the synthetic.

Vitamin K

This fat-soluble vitamin is formed in the intestines. It is necessary in forming the blood-clotting substance prothrombin. Vitamin K can be depleted by X rays, other radiation, mineral oil, antibiotics, and sulfa medications. It often appears on food labels as the additive phytonadione.

Benefits
• Necessary for clotting

Recommended Amount
There is no required recommended daily allowance because vitamin K is made in the intestines (unless there is severe chronic intestinal disease). Small dogs, 15 mcg.; medium dogs, 30 mcg.; large dogs, up to 60 mcg.

Deficiency Symptoms
Poor blood clotting (hypoprothrombinemia).

Advice
Vitamin K deficiency is rare, except in certain diseases. Liver disease can decrease the amount of fat absorbed from the intestine, thus lessening the amount of vitamin K absorbed. Young puppies can have clotting problems of unknown origin in which vitamin K supplementation is required. In any of these cases, consultation with a veterinarian PRIOR to supplementation is important.

If your dog has been on long-term antibiotic therapy, that could decrease the bacterial population necessary to make the vitamin K. Giving a probiotic (yogurt culture-type bacteria) at least two hours before or after the antibiotic will help restore the flora necessary for a healthy intestine as well as for the production of vitamin K.

MINERALS

Vitamins cannot be used by the body without minerals. Minerals must be ingested; they can't be made in the body, as certain vitamins are (C, K, etc.). Mineral supplementation can be tricky because of all the interactions. Excessive supplementation can create havoc.

Calcium

Calcium is a mineral that, along with phosphorus, is required in the dog's diet. Its balance is dependent on phosphorus; there should be approximately equal quantities of the two. Calcium is necessary for strong teeth and bones, and a healthy nervous system. For effective absorption and utilization of calcium, vitamin D must be present.

Benefits

- Promotes growth and maintenance of strong bones and teeth.
- Improves behavior by keeping the nervous system functioning properly.
- Aids in blood clotting

Recommended Amount

There is no simple way to tell you how much calcium is required, since it is based on the diet itself. The AAFCO minimum requirements are 1.1% calcium and 0.9% phosphorus. Supplementation is generally not required because most pet foods contain more than adequate amounts (20–120% over the minimum requirement).

Sources

Dairy products, sardines, green vegetables.

Deficiency Symptoms

Decrease in bone density, limping, aversion to activity, spontaneous fractures (soft bones), rickets in young or old animals, and rubber jaw. Lactating dogs can develop muscle weakness (eclampsia) that could be life-threatening.

Advice

This is one mineral for which old wives' tales certainly don't hold true—don't supplement because you want your dog's bones to grow hard and long, or because you want your dog's ears to stand erect, or because your dog is pregnant!

Oversupplementation can cause all kinds of problems, bone disease being one. Though you may not see it by looking at the dog, damaging effects can occur. While some breeders will add calcium to their dogs' diets and swear that it is not harming their bone development, they don't have X rays to prove that the dogs' bones are in fact healthy! Even though a dog doesn't have obvious signs of bone problems, that doesn't mean the bones are in good health. I've seen X rays of normal-looking dogs supplemented with very small quantities of bone meal, and the bones were not healthy!

If bone disease is not enough to discourage you from supplementing calcium, let's talk about pregnant dogs. During pregnancy the demand for calcium starts to increase about halfway through. Calcium blood levels are regulated by many components that all work together to bring the calcium from the intestines into the blood; from the blood into the bones, growing puppies, or mammary glands; and finally out in the urine if there is too much. When an owner supplements with calcium, the supplementation confuses the body regulatory system, and the body then depends only on the added calcium. If adequate calcium is not being supplied, the mother dog and or her puppies can become hypocalcemic (low calcium) and can die. And last, if you are still intent on adding calcium, you need to know that excess calcium can cause bloat.

If you are really worried about getting enough calcium into your dog or puppy, do it the natural way: feed an extra meal with calcium-rich food, prepare a Dr. Jane calcium delight, or add a scrambled egg or cottage cheese to your dog's food. Make sure that your calcium-rich food doesn't exceed 15% of the total food volume.

Cobalt

Cobalt is essentially a part of vitamin B12 (cobalamin) that's needed for the manufacturing of red blood cells.

Benefits
- Helps prevent anemia

Recommended Amount
.0005 per kg. of body weight for adults. Double that amount for lactation and growth.
.016 mg. for small-medium dogs
.2 mg. for large dog

Sources
Meat, kidney, liver, milk, oysters, and clams.

Deficiency Symptoms
Same as for B12.

Advice
Cobalt is required only when vitamin B12 is deficient. Since strict vegetarians are the only deficient group I know of, keep your dogs as carnivores, the way they should be.

Copper

This mineral is necessary for converting the iron in your dog's body into hemoglobin (the iron-containing pigment in the red blood cells that carry oxygen from the lungs to the tissues). Copper is important for the effective utilization of vitamin C. It is often listed on food labels as the additive copper gluconate or cupric sulfate.

Benefits
- Increases energy and alertness by aiding effective iron absorption

Recommended Amount
The minimum AAFCO requirements depend on the formulation of the food. Dosage for small dogs should not exceed 0.5 mg. daily; large dogs, no more than 2mg. daily.

Sources
Beef, liver, kidney, peas, avocados, dandelion greens, oranges, seafood, soybeans, garlic, lentils.

Deficiency Symptoms
Deficiency can be caused by overzealous supplementation of zinc or iron. Signs of it include bone problems with symptoms similar to lack of calcium, slow growth, dry and brittle coat, pica (eating unusual things), anemia.

Advice
If your dog is eating a food balanced by the manufacturer, there is sufficient copper in it to supply your dog's needs. An excess of copper can create myriad problems, including decreased absorption of other minerals.

There are a few breeds of dogs in which there is a hereditary defect in copper metabolism, causing a build-up of copper in the liver. In Bedlington terriers, Portuguese water dogs, and West Highland white terriers, copper supplementation should be avoided except under the direction of your veterinarian. Dogs with copper storage disease need to avoid foods that contain high amounts of copper. (See section on liver storage disease).

If your dog is anemic, chances are your veterinarian has given you a supplement that contains copper. If you want to, you may add copper-rich foods to the diet.

Iodine

A particularly vital mineral, iodine affects the function of the thyroid gland, which controls metabolism. An undersupply can cause hypothyroidism; an oversupply, hyperthyroidism. It is contained in high quantities in most pet foods.

Benefits
- Promotes normal bone growth

- Aids in weight control by burning excess fat

- Helps prevent and remedy both hypothyroidism and hyperthyroidism

  - Is responsible for your pet's general physical and mental energy

Recommended Amount
The AAFCO minimum requirements are based on the food formulation, and only trace amounts are required.

Sources
Seafood (shrimp, scallops), vegetables grown in iodine-rich soil, kelp, garlic, sea salt, sesame seeds, soybeans, summer squash, turnip greens.

Deficiency Symptoms
Lethargy, slow mental reactions, unexplainable weight gain (hypothyroidism), hair loss without irritation (usually on both sides of the body), dandruff, nervousness, ravenous appetite, enlarged thyroid gland.

Advice
Since dog food has enough iodine in it, you don't have to worry about this mineral unless your pet is in fact hypothyroid because of low iodine levels, or you are feeding large quantities of fruits and vegetables known for their ability to block the use of iodine in the body. Hypothyroid dogs should not have brussels sprouts, cabbage, cauliflower, kale, spinach, turnips, peaches, or pears in large quantities. Kelp contains many micronutrients, including iodine, that can be helpful to a low-functioning thyroid. Since kelp can sometimes worsen hyperthyroid disease, read the label of any supplement you give to your dog, since it can contain kelp. Ask your veterinarian BEFORE supplementing with it.

Iron

Iron is vital to forming hemoglobin in red blood corpuscles, which transport oxygen to body tissues. It is important for the proper metabolization of B vitamins. It is easily available and utilized from meat products as long as the dog has an adequate supply of copper (not too much), cobalt, manganese, and vitamin C.

Benefits
- Improves the immune system and resistance to disease

  - Aids in growth

  - Reduces absorption of lead and helps prevent its harmful effects

  - Cures or prevents iron deficiency anemia

• Necessary to produce hemoglobin, the major oxygen-transporting component of the blood

Recommended Amount
The AAFCO minimum requirements are dependent on the food formulation. If supplementing because of anemia, no more than 10–40 mg. per day is acceptable.

Sources
Eggs, liver, fish, meat, chicken, green leafy vegetables, whole grains, almonds, avocados, beets, blackstrap molasses, brewer's yeast, dates, kelp, lentils, lima beans, parsley, peaches, pears, pumpkins, raisins, rice, wheat bran and soybeans.

Deficiency Symptoms
Brittle coat and nails, fatigue, white gums, weakness, anemia, impaired growth.

Advice
Iron is a very important nutrient. Popeye couldn't have built up all those muscles without it. If you think that your puppy, adult, or senior dog needs iron, have its hemoglobin and red blood cells tested. If tests confirm the need for iron, ask your veterinarian for a tonic that includes other blood builders: B vitamins, folic acid, and vitamin C. Vitamin C can increase the absorption of iron in the body by 30%. Pet Tinic is my favorite tonic. Since iron supplements cause constipation and black stools, you may want to add one of the iron-rich foods to your dog's food 4–5 times weekly (no more than 15%). Brewer's yeast treats contain significant iron. Forget about leafy vegetables; there's just not enough iron available. Puppies can sometimes become weak and anemic, especially if they can't nurse or are stressed. A dab of blackstrap molasses on their tongue every 2–3 hours can be a lifesaver. It gives them iron and energy.

Magnesium

This mineral is important for the proper metabolism and use of vitamins C, E, and B complex, calcium, phosphorous, sodium, and potassium. It is used to convert blood sugar into energy and is essential for nerve and muscle function.

It's very important for bone mineralization and is often combined with calcium and phosphorus in bone supplements. However, it is the prime cause of urinary stone formation.

Benefits

- Helps to regulate the cardiovascular system and body temperature

- Aids in modifying nervous behavior by working with calcium as a natural tranquilizer

- Has been found to help decrease the symptoms of asthma

- Used to combat constipation

Recommended Amount

A reasonable dietary level is about 100–300 mg. Pregnant dogs require additional. The AAFCO minimum requirements for magnesium are calculated according to the rest of the food formula. Supplementation at 100–500 mg daily is safe and effective. It is often listed on food labels as magnesium phosphate or magnesium sulfate.

Sources

Dairy products, fish, meat, sea food, apples, apricots, avocados, bananas, brewer's yeast, garlic, kelp, blackstrap molasses, and whole grains.

Deficiency Symptoms

Retarded growth, spreading of toes and abnormal leg extension, hyperexcitability, convulsions, and bone malformation.

Advice

This is truly an important mineral because of the delicate balance between it and the other minerals, especially calcium and copper. Watch out for oversupplementing so you don't create diarrhea, bone disease, or urinary stones. If you want to make sure that your dog is getting enough, your best bet is to add the natural foods mentioned above. I like to add fresh garlic (cooked or powdered garlic loses many nutrients). Magnesium can be used therapeutically to help promote regularity and to help open the airways in the lungs of asthmatic dogs. Check with your vet. Dosage: 50–75 mg. for a small dog, 100–250 mg. for a medium dog, 250–500 mg. for a large dog.

Manganese

This is an important mineral for bone growth and structure. It is necessary for proper utilization of biotin, and vitamins B1, C, and E, and for fat metabolism. It aids in forming the principal hormone of the thyroid gland (thyroxin). It's needed for a healthy immune and nervous system.

Benefits

- Improves agility and alertness

• Helps alleviate behavior problems by reducing nervousness

• If combined with B vitamins, it helps to give an overall sense of well-being

Recommended Amount

This mineral does all its work in small amounts. Small dogs, 1–2 mg.; medium dogs, 5–10 mg.; large dogs, 15–20mg. The AAFCO minimum requirements are determined by the food formulation.

Deficiency symptoms are rare.

Sources

Avocados, nuts, seaweed, whole grains, egg yolk, and green leafy vegetables.

Advice

If you are feeding a well-balanced dog food, you don't have to worry about supplementing this mineral. If you are creating your dog's meals at home, your general supplement must include this mineral to help prevent reproductive problems and bone disease (short, thick brittle bones). Seaweed is a great supplement that you can add to your homemade diet to make sure it has enough manganese. Most dogs will eat some type of seaweed.

Phosphorus

Phosphorus is the mineral that works with calcium and is indispensable for your dog's diet. It must have an approximately equal amount of calcium to function properly in growth and maintenance of healthy bones, teeth, muscles, and nervous system. Excessive amounts or an incorrect calcium:phosphorous ratio can result in calcium deficiency. It is listed on dog food labels as calcium phosphate, sodium phosphate, or sodium pyrophosphate. Its value can be lessened by too much iron or magnesium.

Benefits

• Increases energy by aiding the metabolism of fats and starches

• Helps healing of bones and other injuries

• Promotes healthier gums and teeth, and growth

Recommended Amount

The amount of phosphorus depends on the amount of calcium and other minerals in the diet. Larger amounts are recommended for pregnant or lactating dogs. The AAFCO minimum requirement is 2.3 gms. per 1,000 calories for a pregnant or lactating dog, and 1.4 gms. for maintenance. A safe supplementation dosage is 50 mg. for small dogs and 300 mg. for large dogs.

Sources
Bone meal, asparagus, oat bran, meat, egg yolk, fish, and garlic.

Deficiency Symptoms
Generally caused by an all-meat diet or excessive calcium supplementation: bone disease, lack of appetite (anorexia), constipation, lameness, loss of teeth.

Advice
Phosphorus is the best example of how complex nutritional supplementation can be. If the ratio of phosphorus to other minerals is wrong, havoc can occur within the dog you love so much! AAFCO's suggested calcium:phosphorus ratio is 1.1–1.4 parts calcium to 1 part phosphorous. I've seen kidney and bone disease as a result of imbalanced home-cooked meals. Depending on the addition of meat and bone meal to balance a primarily meat diet doesn't always work. Reduced phosphorus is extremely important in dogs with kidney disease. (See section on kidney disease).

Potassium

Working with sodium, this mineral regulates your dog's cardiovascular system: heartbeat, fluid balance, and blood pressure. It is essential for nerve impulses to travel through the body from muscle to muscle to spinal cord to brain. It is easily depleted by diarrhea, excessive sugar, diuretics, severe stress, and kidney disease. It is listed on pet food labels as one of the following: potassium chloride, potassium glycerophosphate, or potassium iodide.

Benefits
- Helps improve mental and muscle reflexes

- Aids in allergy treatments and elimination of body wastes

- Can help stimulate appetite

Recommended Amount
The AAFCO minimum requirement is 0.6% of the total food. Supplementation for the average dog is .5–mEq of potassium chloride per pound, or 25 mg. for small dogs, 25–50 mg. for medium dogs, 100 mg. for large and giant.

Sources

Bananas, blackstrap molasses, brewer's yeast, figs, dates, garlic, potatoes, raisins, torula yeast, wheat bran, yams, dairy products, fish, and cantaloupe.

Deficiency Symptoms

Potassium depletion causes general weakness and stiffness. Many chronically ill dogs respond to potassium supplementation. I recommend a potassium supplement for any dog with kidney disease (as long as he is urinating) or diarrhea, regardless of their potassium blood level. Dogs with heart disease generally benefit from potassium as well.

Advice

To increase appetite, add potassium chloride (salt substitute) to the food, ¼ tsp or 1 gram per 15 lbs. of body weight. Combining it with zinc (1 mg. per 3 lbs) and B complex will help ensure its success. For dogs with kidney disease, add salt substitute to the food: 1 gm. daily for small dogs and 5 gm. daily for giant breeds. Make sure that you tell your veterinarian what you are doing, because if your dog is not producing enough urine, you can poison your dog. Your vet has potassium supplements in a gel, powder, or biscuit form. For orphaned puppies with diarrhea, mix Gerber's rice cereal with potassium into their milk substitute formula, or add a pinch of salt substitute to it. Certain dogs form calcium oxalate crystals (dalmatians are notorious for them). Potassium can help dissolve them! Ask your veterinarian for liquid potassium citrate

Quercetin

This natural substance falls under the category of bioflavanoids. Even though they aren't "true" vitamins, they are sometimes called vitamin P because they cannot be produced by the body. An antioxidant, bioflavanoids work synergistically with vitamin C. They are found just below the peel of citrus fruits and some other foods.

Benefits

- Increases the use of vitamin C in the body.

- Improves circulation

- Decreases inflammation due to allergies

- Helps to relieve pain from sprains, strains, and bruises

Recommended Amount

Large dogs, 500–1000 mg. daily; medium dogs, 250–500 mg. daily; small dogs, 100–200 mg. daily.

Sources

Beneath the peel of apricots, cherries, grapefruit, grapes, lemons, oranges, prunes, and rose hips. It's also in buckwheat and peppers. Tablets and capsules are available from health food stores.

Deficiency Symptoms

Possible vitamin C-like deficiency symptoms, such as inflammation of the gums, bleeding of small vessels, cataract formation.

Advice

This extraordinary antioxidant is truly an allergic animal's best anti-inflammatory nutrient. It is expensive, so start with low doses and work up to the recommended amount. Give your dog 2–3 weeks to adjust to the low dosage before increasing it. Too much too soon can cause diarrhea. It is usually combined with vitamin C and bromelain (an enzyme). Because it tastes slightly bitter, you may have to disguise it well in food.

Selenium

Once thought to be very toxic, selenium is a vital antioxidant that generally needs to be supplemented. It helps keep the heart muscle healthy, and works in combination with vitamin E to ensure a healthy immune system. It's necessary for the pancreas to function correctly.

Benefits

- Combined with vitamin E, it aids in antibody formation
- A powerful antioxidant that helps fight "free radical" damage
- Helps to prevent cataracts
- Useful in treating enlarged prostates

Recommended Amount

Overdosing is easy to do with this mineral. No more than 25 mcg. for small dogs and 100 mcg. for giant dogs.

Sources

Brewer's yeast, dairy products, garlic, molasses, onions, seafood, torula yeast, and wheat germ.

Deficiency Symptoms

Breakdown of muscles, including the heart muscle, and bone disease.

Advice

This mineral is currently under surveillance as a cancer fighter and chronic disease fighter. Not as toxic as it was thought to be, it is so essential in the antioxidant pathways that it must be included in any antioxidant mixture.

Sodium

Sodium (salt) works with potassium to regulate fluid balance, muscle contraction, and nerve stimulation. It is necessary for nerves and muscles to function, and must be balanced with potassium.

Benefits

- Helps keep reflexes at optimal performance

- Aids in preventing heat prostration

- Regulates cardiovascular function, including blood pressure

Recommended Amount

The minimum AAFCO requirements, based on the food formulation, are 0.3% for growth and lactation and .06% for maintenance; they are probably too high.

Sources

Table salt, sea salt (my preference), shellfish, kidney, beets, bacon.

Deficiency Symptoms

Deficiencies are rare, except when heat or extreme exercise causes excessive loss of water and salt. Symptoms include pica (eating strange things), fatigue, and slow growth.

Advice

This is another mineral that is helpful for managing certain medical problems. For struvite crystals or stones, add ¼ tsp. of salt per 12 lbs. of body weight to the dog's food. Hills Prescription S/D is presalted food for dissolution of these crystals. Make sure that your dog has unlimited access to fresh water. For heart disease, you should restrict the sodium only when your dog is diagnosed as having it, not just because it is old. There are veterinary-only diets by Hills, Purina, and Waltham that are well-balanced and have low amounts of sodium. There is no such thing as a dog food without it. Snacks must not have any salt added to them or be naturally salty. Dogs can get high blood pressure—and since most of the commercial dog foods are already high in salt, check the ingredients in all of your treats. Make sure that salt is not one.

Zinc

A top-notch major mineral, zinc is necessary for protein synthesis, development of reproductive organs, contractility of the muscles, and tissue growth. It is easily destroyed in food processing, which is why it needs to be added. On dog food labels it is often listed as the additive zinc oxide or zinc sulfate. Zinc is important for reproductive organs, both female and male, and essential for a healthy immune system and the utilization of vitamin E. It also interacts with calcium and copper.

Benefits

• Aids in healing burns, sores, flea bites, and fractures

• Helps to maintain a healthy skin and coat

• Supports the antioxidants vitamin E, beta carotene, vitamin C, and selenium

• Increases immune functions

• Useful for many skin conditions (dandruff, hot spots, dermatitis)

• Helps in managing diabetic dogs

• Essential in combating prostate disease

• Improves appetite

• Helps protect the liver

Recommended Amount

1–2 mg. per pound is the general supplemental dosage. Oversupplementation will cause calcium and copper deficiency.

Sources

Brewer's yeast, torula yeast, beef, pork, lamb, egg yolk, and sardines.

Advice

This is truly a wonder mineral. If you are giving your dog antioxidants (vitamins C and E, beta-carotene, and selenium), zinc should be part of that combination. Huskies, malamutes, and other northern breeds can develop skin problems around the eyes if zinc is not added to their diets. If you have a dog with copper storage disease, zinc is a must, 3 to 6 times daily, not to exceed the above recommended amount per day. As an appetite stimulator, combine it with B vitamins and potassium.

Deficiency Symptoms

Retarded growth, smaller sized adult, coarse coat, skin lesion (especially around the eye in huskies, malamutes, and other north breeds), weight loss, conjunctivitis and a poor immune system.

Herbs, Grasses and Other Natural Supplements

Believe it or not, modern medicine and pharmaceuticals are relatively new; they didn't get started until the early 1900s. Prior to that, dating back to early man, remedies were made from naturally occurring substances. It's not hard to imagine our ancestors watching sick animals as they ate the plants needed to get well, and their own experimentation with plants and foodstuffs for their health problems. Generation by generation, natural remedies became refined, plants used for medicinal purposes became known as herbs, and eventually herbal remedies were included in physicians' books: what they should be used for, dosages, etc.

If herbs are so beneficial, you are probably asking, why did we turn from them to drugs (derived from the Middle English word *droggs*, which was used when talking about healers drying herbs). The problems with herbal and natural medicines are time, efficacy, taste, and side effects. Most herbs need to be taken frequently—certainly more often than most pharmaceuticals—have unpleasant tastes, and can have side effects that include death!

Digitalis is an excellent example of why drugs became the norm for medicine. Derived from a very poisonous herb, digitalis is dosed so that side effects are less apt to occur than with the whole herb; is given in a small tablet; and is given only once daily. One by one, herbs were replaced by man-made products; an estimated 20% of all our drugs are derived from plants.

Today, people want to go back to the whole food, natural approach to healing. Pharmaceutical companies are sending scientists into the jungles to locate herbs and other beneficial plants. You don't have to travel anywhere to start using natural medicine—you can start right here. If you can't find some of these items at your local health food store, try the Animal's Apawthecary, (800) 822-9609.

ACIDOPHILUS

Sour milk and yogurt are known for their acidophilus content. Acidophilus are bacteria, *Lactobacillus acidophilus*. A healthy dog's intestines contain a large amount of these friendly, necessary bacteria that keep the harmful bacteria under control.

Benefits

• Helpful in control of diarrhea, especially after antibiotic use or parasite load

• Helps to keep the intestinal cells healthy

• Keeps the intestinal bacteria population balanced

• Helps with the digestion of food

Recommended Amount

One billion units for small and medium dogs and two billion for large and giant dogs. It is best taken on an empty stomach an hour before eating, or at least 2 hours after eating, but it is still effective if combined with food. Don't give it at the same time you give antibiotics. Space it 3–4 hours before or after.

Sources

• Acidophilus is naturally present in fermented dairy products such as buttermilk, yogurt, kefir, and cheese.

• It is available in health food stores and pet shops as a liquid, powder, or capsule. Most forms have to be refrigerated except for Kyo-Dophilus.

Deficiency Symptoms

Diarrhea, mucus in the stools, gas, unthriftiness (shaggy coat, dry skin, no energy, no sparkle in the eyes).

Advice

A normal dog should have enough acidophilus in its intestinal tract. Antibiotics, intestinal parasites, or any chronic intestinal problem require a supplement. These bacteria, combined with other friendly ones, are essential for the intestinal cells to stay healthy. Healthy intestinal cells are very important, especially in young puppies and older dogs. Healthy intestines provide a barrier, keeping the wrong things from entering the blood and circulating around the body. We all know how dogs seem to eat anything: garbage, feces, nondigested foods, etc. If harmful bacteria are swallowed, and the intestinal cells are not healthy, the bacteria could enter the blood and cause illness. Your dog has a greater chance of developing food allergies if its food is not totally digested, and enters the bloodstream in that state because the intestinal barrier is not healthy. If puppies are weaned before the intestinal barrier is formed, the chances that they'll develop food allergies increase.

ALFALFA

Alfalfa is one of the richest mineral foods because of its deep roots. It contains many nutrients, including calcium, magnesium, phosphorus, potassium, selenium, chlorophyll, and all known vitamins.

Benefits

- A well-balanced multinutrient antioxidant
- Alone or in combination with other herbs, a treatment for arthritis
- Helps fight bad breath
- Helps detoxify the liver

Recommended Amount

Depending on the freshness of your alfalfa and its purity (sometimes it's mixed with fillers or other substances), dosages will vary. A large dog can be given the amount recommended for humans. A medium or small dog should get a proportion of that amount.

Sources

- Health food stores and mail-order herbal catalogs

- Animal's Apawthecary, (800) 822-9609, for alfalfa tinctures made with glycerin, for better taste

Advice

As with any additive, start with a little and gradually work up to the recommended dosage.

BEE POLLEN

A fine, powderlike material found on the anthers of flowering plants and gathered by bees. It is claimed to be one of the oldest complete foods in the world, with over 75 nutrients. Its sweet/sour taste generally appeals to dogs.

Benefits

- A natural antibiotic
- Promotes a healthy immune system
- Useful in alleviating allergy symptoms

Recommended Amount

Recommended dosage will vary, depending on the manufacturer. The usual adult dosage can be used for a large dog. Medium and small dogs get proportionately less.

Sources

Health food stores, health product catalogs

Advice

Dogs with allergies to airborne substances can be allergic to pollen. However, bee pollen is different from the pollen that blows in the air. If your dog has airborne allergies, chances are that bee pollen can help reduce the symptoms. Just start very slowly to make sure there are no reactions.

Containing anywhere from 10 to 35% protein, B complex vitamins, fatty acids, enzymes, natural hormones, minerals, and other vitamins, bee pollen is a naturally complete nutritional supplement that will not interfere with the balance of dog food. Because it has such a wide array of nutrients, it often can help restore the natural balance of the body; thus I prefer this as your "one a day" multivitamin-mineral supplement rather than a synthetic one. Diabetic and hypoglycemic animals should not be given bee pollen because of the sugar content.

CHAMOMILE

Known as *Anthemis nobilis*, an herb also called "big plant," chamomile has beneficial medicinal properties.

Benefits

• Helpful in diarrhea or upset stomach

• The tea can be made into an a eye wash for irritated eyes

• Can be used alone or with other natural remedies for relief of nervousness

• Can be used in a vaporizer for relief of lung and nasal congestion

Recommended Amount

As a tincture (ask for one without alcohol), 1–10 drops in the water dish (depending on dog's size) or directly into the mouth 2–3 times daily. As a tea, add 1–2 teaspoons or 1–2 tea bags to one cup boiling water, ¼–1 full tsp. honey, cover, and let sit for 3–5 minutes. Filter.

Sources

Health food stores, supermarkets, and herbal catalogs

Advice

This is known for its fragrant aromatic scent, so it's important to cover your teas so that the vapors don't dissapate. Since it is pleasant tasting, the addition of honey is not essential.

DANDELION

Taraxacum densleonis, also called lion's tooth or white endive, dandelion has beneficial medicinal properties; it is rich in iron, B vitamins, sulfur, zinc, and many nutritive salts.

Benefits

• Useful in weight loss programs

• Useful in treating anemia

• A natural diuretic

• Liver detoxifier

Recommended Amount

For weight loss, chop up fresh dandelion or add fresh dry dandelion to your dog's food daily: ¼– ½ tsp. for small dogs, 2 tbsp. for giant breeds. For anemia or for kidney disease (to promote urination), use the tincture, 2–6 drops twice daily, or follow the recommended adult dosage for large dogs, decreasing the amount given proportionately with the dog's size.

Sources

- Fresh produce stores, during the season
- Health food stores for tinctures or dried
- Animal's Apawthecary for better-tasting tinctures, (800) 822-9609

Advice

If feeding fresh dandelion leaf, the centre rib of *young* leaves are not that bitter. I like to boil dandelion leaf along with spinach, sprinkle with salt and minced garlic and add it to the dog food. When using the tincture be sure to use the glycerin preserved rather than the alcohol. The glycerin helps mask the bitterness of the herb.

ECHINACEA

Known as *Echinacea angustifolia* or purple coneflower, echinacea is very bitter but has beneficial medicinal properties. It is known as an antibacterial, antiviral herb.

Benefits

- Builds the immune system
- Can be used instead of antibiotics

Recommended Amount

As a tincture, 2–8 drops every 4 hrs. (or recommended adult dosage for the large dog, decreasing amount given proportionately to smaller size) during the first 3 days, then to three to four times daily. Don't use this herb for longer than 3 weeks, or in conjunction with antibiotics.

Sources

- Health food stores and herbal catalogs
- Animal's Apawthecary for better-tasting herbs, (800) 822-9609

Advice

This is a powerful alternative to antibiotics, which are limited in their usage. For one thing, they act ONLY on bacteria, and are ineffective against viral infections that are so common in dogs. While antibiotics will eliminate the problem if it is bacterial in nature, they do nothing to prevent recurrent or future infections. Common puppy diseases such as pyoderma (pimples on the inner thighs), kennel cough, ear infections, and eye infections generally respond to this herb, which works by boosting the immune system. Thus it not only fights off the invader but also reinforces the body's defense so it doesn't return.

GARCINIA CAMBOGIA

A yellow fruit native to India that is used in cooking (curry) there, *Garcina* is used to curb hunger, increase energy levels, and calm indigestion. It's commonly called Citrimax.

Benefits

- Decreases begging
- Helps burn calories
- Increases metabolism
- Digestive aid

Recommended Amount

Large dogs, 500 mg. before each meal; medium dogs, 250 mg. before each meal; small dogs, 75–125 mg. before each meal.

Sources

Natural product catalogs and health food stores. It usually comes in capsules, but you may be able to find a chewable form for dogs in a pet store that carries natural products.

Advice

Garcina cambogia is very popular among dieters because it can be combined with all types of substances, including caffeine and other stimulants. Make sure your product contains *only* the herb. Since it will decrease your dog's appetite, the optimum way to give it is directly by mouth an hour before meals. You can also open the capsule and put the appropriate amount directly into the food. Referred to as the "couch potato's magical herb," it both revitalizes and reduces the dog.

GARLIC

Garlic is a member of the lily family, and has long been used both for taste and for its medicinal properties. Described as a natural antibiotic/antiparasitic substance, it contains potassium, which is useful for treating kidney disease and old age.

Benefits

- Strengthens the immune system
- Enhances flavor of food (garlic powder)
- Helps promote healthy skin and coat (garlic oil)
- Combined with brewer's yeast, may repel fleas
- Blood thinning agent and a cardiovascular tonic
- May have anticancer effects
- Decreases blood sugar

Recommended Amount

To make your own garlic oil, wet 2 or 3 cloves of garlic with vodka and crush them. Add them to 4 oz. olive oil, and shake it vigorously. Leave it in the refrigerator for at least an hour. Add ½ to 1 tsp. of the oil per pound of food, 3 to 4 times weekly. (The oil, covered, will stay fresh about a month in the refrigerator.) If you're using fresh garlic, feed ¼–1 chopped clove per meal, 3 or 4 times weekly.

Sources

Produce stores, health food stores, natural product catalogs

Advice

Too much garlic can cause internal bleeding, anemia, gas, or upset stomach. I don't recommend the use of garlic for anemic dogs, dogs with any type of bleeding disorder, or puppies under six weeks of age (they can tend to be anemic). Cooking destroys garlic's medicinal qualities, so if you sauté garlic for your dog, other than taste, it's not doing much.

KELP

Kelp is one of the 2,500 different types of seaweed. It is rich in vitamins, minerals, and trace elements, and contains a natural blend of antioxidants. It's known for its iodine content, which varies with the type of seaweed but can be 5–10 times the amount found in iodized salt.

Benefits

- Supplies the body with iodine, necessary for proper thyroid functioning

- A great multinutrient supplement

- Useful in thyroid, heart, kidney, bladder, and reproductive diseases

- Useful in the control of arthritis

- Better skin and coat

- Weight control

- An internal supplement for flea control

Recommended Amount

The potency of kelp will vary from manufacturer to manufacturer. Generally, one drop of liquid kelp daily for small dogs, and 3–4 drops daily for giant breeds.

Sources

- Health food stores and herbal catalogs

Advice

While kelp can be miraculous, it has its disadvantages. It should not be used in dogs with heart disease or high blood pressure. I recommend its use only in dogs with low thyroid (hypothyroidism) or older dogs whose thyroid function tests are normal but have gained weight, have dandruff and/or poor coat, and basically act like couch potatoes.

VALERIAN

Its scientific name is *Valeriana officinalis*, and it's otherwise known as "all-heal." Only the root is used in herbal medicine.

Benefits

- Antianxiety, used in place of tranquilizers
- Useful to relieve muscle cramping
- Painkiller
- Useful to help control epileptic fits

Recommended Amount

As a tincture (without alcohol), the usual dosage for a large dog is 2–4 drops in food or directly in the mouth 2–3 hrs. prior to the anticipated stressful event. It can be repeated once more during the stressful event. Tinctures, capsules, and teas will vary in their potency. A large dog can be given the recommended adult dosage; a small dog, a suggested child's dose.

Sources

- Health food stores and herbal catalogs
- Animal's Apawthecary for better-tasting herbs, (800) 822-9609

Advice

This is a very bitter herb, so for picky dogs, you will have to disguise it before giving it. Even though valerian is very safe, too much can cause an upset stomach. I recommend using it for dogs who are afraid of thunder and lightning, and for those with separation anxiety and other types of nervousness.

VEGETABLE DIGESTIVE ENZYMES

Derived from plants, these enzymes break down food into basic building blocks that the body can use. There are different types of digestive enzymes, all of them part of the protein family. There are four basic groups: lipase, which breaks down fats; protease, which breaks down protein; amylase, which breaks down starch; and cellulase, which breaks down fiber.

Benefits

- Increases digestion of all foods
- Useful in dogs with gas
- Reduces fecal volume
- Increases overall body health

Recommended Amount

Dosage will vary with the type of enzyme and the manufacturer. Generally, the human dosage would be used for large dogs and decreased in proportion for smaller ones.

Sources

- Health food stores and herbal catalogs
- Prozyme (800) 522-5537

Advice

Canned and dry dog foods are processed, so the natural enzymes in the ingredients have been destroyed. I recommend the addition of vegetable enzymes to any food to ensure that the dog gets the most from its food. Generally speaking, no matter what type of problem your dog may have, increased nutrition is indicated. If your dog is a rapid eater; is unthrifty; has digestive problems, skin disease, or a chronic disease; or is a senior, add these enzymes to the food. Vegetable enzymes are not the same as those derived from animals. The addition of vegetable enzymes to any type of dog food will not unbalance its careful formulation.

Recipes

Dr. Jane's Calcium Delight

Use this as a supplemental meal for pregnant dogs or for puppies.

1 soft-boiled egg
1 pinch of salt
1 bowl cooked oatmeal
¼ c. lactose-free milk

½ tsp. honey
½ tsp. wheat germ
2 strips cooked bacon (optional)

Combine all the ingredients in a bowl. Mix well and serve.

(Note: For adult large and giant dogs use 1¾ cups water to 1 cup of oatmeal. This will yield two servings. For adult small to medium dogs use 1 cup of water and ½ cup of oatmeal. This will yield one serving. For puppies mix ½ cup water with ¼ cup oats to yield ½ serving.)

Dr. Jane's Slurpy

Use this as a protein energy booster for puppies; pregnant or lactating dogs; dogs recovering from surgery; or debilitated dogs.

¼ c. goat's milk (cow's milk is
   acceptable)
⅛–1 tbsp. corn oil
¼–2 tsp. of honey

¼–1 banana
Pinch of salt
⅛–1 tsp. wheat germ
Cream of Wheat

Put honey and milk into a saucepan and heat until the honey becomes fluid. Add the Cream of Wheat, sprinkling a little at a time until the mixture becomes slightly thickened. Remove the pan from the burner and add banana, oil, and salt. Sprinkle with wheat germ and serve it (make sure the slurpy is not too hot). This can be given in between meals once or twice daily, or before bed. Depending on the size of your dog, adjust quantities accordingly. The smallest amounts are for small dogs, and the largest amounts are for large dogs. Keep remainder in refrigerator in a sealed container. Microwave to warm but be sure to stir and *not* overheat it. It can be left in the refrigerator for 3 days only. Don't add the wheat germ to the "Batch"; rather, sprinkle it on when used.

GARLIC DOG BISCUITS

These are an excellent substitute for store-bought treats that can be full of sugar, colors, and preservatives.

1½ c. unbleached flour	⅛ tsp. minced garlic
1½ c. whole wheat flour	1 egg, slightly beaten
½ c. cornmeal	1–1¼ c. water
⅛ c. nonfat dry milk	

Stir together the first 3 ingredients in a large bowl. Add the remaining ingredients, with just enough water that the dough is stiff. Knead the dough until it becomes smooth, then roll it out ¼" thick. Using a bone-shaped cookie cutter, cut out biscuits. Place them on a lightly greased cookie sheet. Bake in a preheated 350-degree oven for approximately 45 minutes, until golden brown. Shut off the oven and leave biscuits inside for 4 hrs. or more, until hard. Store in an airtight container.

CHICKEN LIVERS A LA CANINE

This dish is a natural protein, vitamin A and D, and iron supplement.

1 lb. chicken livers	Pinch of salt
1⅓ c. whole wheat flour	3 tbsp. of cooking oil
2 eggs, well beaten	

Beat the eggs in a bowl. Add the salt. Immerse the chicken livers in the egg so they are well covered with it. Put the flour into a bag along with the livers. Shake the bag so that all the livers are covered with flour. Store in the refrigerator 1–6 hrs. When ready to fry the livers, add enough oil to cover the bottom of the frying pan. Let the oil heat, then add the livers. Cook at medium heat. Turn the livers as they become medium brown. Take them out of the pan and let them cool. They will stay fresh in the refrigerator for 3–4 days. Warm them in the microwave before giving them as treats.

PUPPY FORMULA

Use this formula as a substitute for mom's milk for newborn puppies if she is missing or unable to feed on her own. These ingredients should be available from your health food store.

3¼ cups fresh cow's milk	4 tsp. citric acid
¾ cup fresh cream	1000 IU vitamin A
1 egg yolk	500 IU vitamin D
1½ tsp bone meal	

If you are feeding a homemade formula exclusively, it's a good idea to give each puppy a small amount of a malt-based vitamin–mineral supplement daily. Nutricall is an old-time favorite.

DR. JANE'S HOME-COOKED FOOD ELIMINATION DIET

Serve this diet for suspected food allergies.

¼ lb. cooked, ground rabbit or lamb	1½ tsp. dicalcium phosphate
1 c. cooked brown rice	
1 tsp. vegetable oil	

Combine all ingredients and mix well. Yields ⅔ lb (300 gm), 795 cal.
　Note: This diet is not balanced and is not meant for longer than 4 weeks.

HIGHLY DIGESTIBLE, LOW RESIDUE DIET

Serve this as an extended remedy for diarrhea after your vet has ruled out illness. See p. 57. When stools return to normal, switch to a low-residue, veterinarian-only diet.

½ c. farina (cooked to make 2 c.)	1 tbsp. corn oil
1½ c. creamed cottage cheese	1 tsp. salt
1 large hard-boiled egg	1 tsp. dicalcium phosphate (salt
2 tbsp. brewer's yeast	substitute)
3 tbsp. warmed honey or blackstrap molasses	1 tsp. calcium carbonate

Cook the farina per instructions on the package, adding the honey or mo-lasses while stirring. Let it cool and add the other ingredients. It yields 2.2 lb. (485 cal). You can feed this diet for 4 weeks max.

Two-Day-Only, Low-Residue Diet

Use 4 parts cooked white or brown rice (4 c.) to 1 part cooked lean meat (boiled chicken, low-fat fish, lean chopped beef, or chopped turkey). Com-bine the rice and meat, adding a pinch of salt. The addition of coconut milk to make the food just a little soupy is optional. This recipe will feed a dog weighing approximately 30 lbs.

Home-Made Diet for Kidney Disease

Even though this diet is balanced and could be fed long-term, it will not lead to optimum health and should be replaced with a veterinary-only kid-ney diet after a period of five to seven days.

¼ lb. ground beef (do not use lean)   3 slices white bread, crumbled
1 large hard-boiled egg   1 tsp. calcium carbonate
2 c. cooked rice

Brown the meat, retaining the fat. Add all the other ingredients and mix, pouring in enough water to make the mixture loose. 750 calories.

Small to medium dog = 1 serving
Large dog = double amts.

Pet Food Manufacturers

If you want to go beyond what's on the label of the food you're serving your dog, call the manufacturer. Don't be shy—your dog's nutritional foundation depends upon the responses to the following questions.

QUESTIONS TO ASK

1. How many veterinarians and nutritionists do you have on staff? May I have their names?

2. Do you have testing facilities on the premises? How many colonies of dogs do you have, and what type? (Some manufactures feed and test their food only on beagles, while others use different breeds and mixes. Since all dogs are different, I prefer a melting pot of breeds.)

3. Do you fund university studies? If so, which ones, and where?

4. Do you publish nutritional papers or books?

5. What is the total digestibility of the dog food? (Since everything that goes in should not come out, the more digestible the food, the better. Supermarket foods generally have digestibilities of 70–80%, while quality alternative foods can go as high as 85–90 plus%).

6. What is the protein digestibility of the dog food? (The more digestible the protein, the better.)

7. What is the caloric density of the food? (You should know how many calories there are in a can, cup, or pound.)

8. Were the calories figured out by using numbers, or were the dogs put into metabolic energy cages where their urine and feces were collected? (Manufacturers that figure calories by using numbers may be taking the easy, more economical way out.)

9. What other type of testing is done besides AAFCO feeding protocols? Kidney and liver function tests? Bone growth studies? Any others?

10. What parts of the meat, chicken, or poultry by-products are used in the food? (If the protein digestibility is high, chances are the by-products and other meats are high-quality.)

PET FOOD MANUFACTURERS' PHONE NUMBERS

Alpo	(800) 366-6033
Bil Jac Foods	(800) 321-1002
Blue Seal Feeds	(800) 367-2730
Federal Foods	(800) 325-6331
Friskies Pet Care/ Friskies Food	(800) 682-7217
Fromm	(800) 867-6547
Happy Jack	(800) 326-5225
Hills Pet Products	(800) 445-5777
Iams	(800) 525-4267
Joy	(800) 245-4125
Kal Kan Foods	(800) 525-5273
Merit Dog Foods	(800) 265-6323
Mighty Dog	no toll free number available
Nabisco	(800) NABISCO
Natural Life Pet Products	(800) 367-2391
Nature's Recipe	(800) 843-4008
Nutra Max, Nutra Products	(800) 833-5330
Old Mother Hubbard Feed Company	(800) 225-0904
Pedigree (Kalkan)	(800) 525-5273
Pet Specialties	(800) 722-3631
Precise Pet Products	(800) 446-7148
Pro Plan, Division of Ralston Purina	(800) 688-PETS
Ralston Purina	(800) 688-PETS
Quaker Oats/Ken-L-Ration	(800) 4MY-PETS
Science Diet	(800) 445-5777

Sensible Choice	(800) 592-6687
Triumph Pet Industries	(800) 331-5144
Vet's Choice Select Balance	(800) 494-PETS
Waltham	(800) 525-5273

Problem/Solution Quick Reference Guide

This section is designed to direct you to additional information for general health problems. All you have to do is look up the problem(s) listed under their subject headings and seek their solution in the appropriate pages of this book.

ATTITUDE (LETHARGY AND APATHY)

POSSIBLE DIET PROBLEM	SOLUTION
Poor quality food, or not recommended amount	Food, pages 21–23, 32
Food is too low in fat, even if your dog is dieting	Food, p. 63; see also Omega-33 fatty acids, p. 45
Not absorbing enough nutrients and/or requires more than in the food	Digestive enzymes, p. 145, bee pollen, p. 139 wheat or oat grass, algae, or vitamin–mineral supplements, p. 43

ALLERGIES

POSSIBLE DIET PROBLEM	SOLUTION
Food sensitivity or allergic response	Food, p. 22–26; Allergy, p. 49
Requires nutritional support for the immune system and to decrease symptoms.	Omega-3 fatty acids, p. 45 Vitamins/minerals, p. 45; Herbs, p. 136; Recipe, p. 147

BAD BREATH

POSSIBLE DIET PROBLEM	SOLUTION
Deficiency of B vitamins in diet	B vitamins, pages 47, 108–115
Poor digestion	Digestive enzymes, p. 145; Acidophilus, p. 137
Requires more or a different type of fiber in the diet	Fiber, p. 10
Tooth and gum disease	See Chewing, p. 54; Vitamin C, pages 116–119 See Nutrional FAQs, p. 99

BLOAT

POSSIBLE DIET PROBLEM	SOLUTION
Too much calcium	Calcium, p. 122
Eating too fast	Mealtime mistakes, pages 36–38; Bloat, p. 73
Poor-quality food	Food, pages 22–26
Impaired digestion	Vegetable enzymes, p. 145
Wrong feeding habits	Right way to feed, pages 37–38

CONSTIPATION

POSSIBLE DIET PROBLEM	SOLUTION
Not enough fiber in diet	Fiber, p. 10
Poor-quality food	Food, pages 22–26

Avoid bones
Incomplete digestion of food   Digestive enzymes, p. 145
If older dog, may need additional   Vitamins–minerals
nutrients, especially B vitamins   pages 119–135

Coprophagy (Eating Feces)

Possible Diet Problem	Solution
Poor-quality food	Food, pages 22–24
Inadequate nutrients	Supplementaion, pages 40, 41, 42
Improper digestion	Digestive Enzymes, p. 145
Puppy habit	FAQs, p. 104
Hunger due to lack of food	

Crusting Around Eyes or Mouth

Possible Diet Problem	Solution
Zinc deficiency, especially sled dog breeds	Zinc, pages 134–135
B vitamin deficiencies	B vitamins, pages 108–115

Diabetes Mellitus

Possible Diet Solutions

Difficult to manage if diet is wrong. Use high-fiber, high-quality
protein, low-fat food.
Vitamin B supplementation, p. 47
Antioxidant supplementation, pages 43, 46
Vitamin/Mineral supplementation, p. 43
No sugars
No change in food or time of feeding
Chromium; 50 mg. for large dogs, 25 mg. for medium dogs, 15
mg. for small dogs

Diarrhea

Possible Diet Problem	Solution
Overindulging in table scraps, particularly fatty meats	Table scraps, p. 36

Too many cereals in the food and or poor food digestibility	Food, pages 5, 10, 22 Digestive enzymes
Eating garbage or spicy, people food, etc.	Don't allow it
Insufficient fiber in diet	Fiber, pages 9, 10
Sensitivity to food or food additive	Allergy, pages 49–50
Intestinal bacterial flora unbalanced	Acidophilus, p. 137
Too much fat in diet/or not enough fat, without enough support nutrients	Fat, pages. 11–12
Rancid or decayed food	
Supplements added too rapidly	
Radical change in diet	

DRY, BRITTLE, OR DULL COAT; DRY SKIN WITH OR WITHOUT FLAKING

POSSIBLE DIET PROBLEM	SOLUTION
Poor-quality food	Food, pages. 10, 22
Needs additional protein	Protein, pages, 7–9
Needs supplement containing B vitamins, proteins, and other helpful nutrients	Brewer's yeast, p. 47 Vitamins–minerals, pages. 41, 43, 47
Requires more fat in the diet	Fat, p. 45; Fatty acid supplements
Needs kelp and tyrosine to stimulate thyroid	Hypothyroid, pages 58, 144

EAR PROBLEMS (CHRONIC EAR DISEASE)

POSSIBLE DIET PROBLEM	SOLUTION
Allergy	Allergy, pages 49–50 Omega-3 fatty acids, p. 45
Poor immune system	Herbs, pages 138, 139, 141, 142, 143 Vitamins C and E, pages 116–122

Excessive Shedding and/or Scanty Coat

Possible Diet Problem	Solution
Needs kelp and tyrosine to stimulate thyroid	Hypothyroid, pages 58, 144
Poor-quality food	Food, pages 22–24; broad vitamin–mineral supplement, pages 43–45
Needs additional nutrients	Digestive enzymes, p. 145; Whole natural food (bee pollen, seaweed), pages, 139, 144
Needs additional protein	Protein, pages 7–9; Brewer's yeast, p. 47
All-meat syndrome	Feeding mistakes, p. 103

Heart Disease

Possible Diet Solutions

Restrict salt
Vitamin B supplementation pages 47, 108–115
High-quality diet pages 22–25
Dandelion, p. 140, 141
L-carnitine: 800–1200 mg. for giant and large breeds; 400–700 mg. for medium breeds; 100–250 mg. for small breeds.
Easy exercise, if any
No excessive weight

Kidney Disease

Possible Diet Solutions

High-quality protein, average amounts unless otherwise advised by veterinarian, pages 7–9
Potassium supplements, p. 131
Vitamin B supplement, pages 47, 108, 115
Restrict phosphorus and calcium
Omega-3 fatty acids, p. 45
Fresh water
Dandelion, p. 140

LACK OF APPETITE

POSSIBLE DIET PROBLEM   SOLUTION

POSSIBLE DIET PROBLEM	SOLUTION
Spoiled dog	FAQs, pages 101, 102 Mealtime mistakes, pages 31, 32
B vitamin deficiencies	B vitamins, p. 47, 108–115
Food not odorous enough for old dog	Mealtimes, p. 37

LACK OF MUSCLE TONE

POSSIBLE DIET PROBLEM	SOLUTION
Calcium deficiency	Calcium, p. 123
Poor quality diet	Food, pages 22, 32, 40, 41
Inadequate utilization of nutrients	Vegetable enzymes, p. 145
L-carnitine deficiency	L-carnitine, p. 46
Insufficient or poor-quality protein	Protein, pages 7, 8, 9,

LAMENESS, LIMPING

POSSIBLE DIET PROBLEM	SOLUTION
Overfeeding puppy or young adult	Mealtimes, p. 36, 59
Oversupplementation, particularly of calcium, vitamin D, or vitamin C when young	Vitamins, pages 40, 41, 123, 124

LIVER DISEASE

POSSIBLE DIET SOLUTIONS

Avoid meat diets
Feed low-residue diets, adding cottage cheese
Low fat
No shellfish or meat by-products
Small amounts of food 4–6 times daily
Vegetable enzymes, p. 145
B vitamin supplementation, pages 47, 108–115
Vitamin C, pages 116, 117, 119

Vitamins A and E, pages 106, 120, 121
Zinc, pages 134–135
Avoid any supplement with copper

OILY SKIN AND OR COAT, RANCID ODOR

POSSIBLE DIET PROBLEM	SOLUTION
Poor-quality food/imbalanced diet	Food, pages 10, 22, 40, 41
Too much fat in diet, probably without enough support nutrients	Fat, pages 11, 12
Insufficient vitamin E and biotin	Vitamins, pages 115, 120, 121
Thyroid problems	Kelp, pages 58, 144

PICA (EATING STRANGE THINGS: DIRT, ROCKS)

POSSIBLE DIET PROBLEM	SOLUTION
Poor-quality diet	Food, pages 22–23, 32
Inadequate nutrients	Supplements, p. 40; Digestive enzymes, p. 145; Herbs, pages 137–145
Needs more fiber	Fiber, pages 19, 20, 55
Improper digestion	Digestive enzymes, p. 145
Hunger due to dieting, wrong food, or infrequent feedings	Food, pages 28, 29, 30 Obesity, pages 62–71

RUNNY EYES

POSSIBLE DIET PROBLEM	SOLUTION
Insufficient vitamins A, E	Vitamins, pages 106, 107, 120, 121
Poor immune system	Herbs, pages 138–139, 141, 143 Vitamins, pages 47,116–122
Allergy	Allergy, pages 49, 50

SPLIT NAILS (SEE UNHEALTHY WHISKERS)

STIFFNESS GETTING UP/WALKING

POSSIBLE DIET PROBLEM	SOLUTION
Poor-quality food	Food, pages 22–24, 32
Insufficient antioxidants	Antioxidants, pages 43, 46
Needs specific nutrients for bone and muscle/arthritis/ hip dysplasia	Zinc, Phosphorous, Zinc, Glucosamine, p. 53
Obesity	Weight Loss Diet Plan, pages 62–71

UNHEALTHY WHISKERS (SHORT, BROKEN, THIN)

POSSIBLE DIET PROBLEM	SOLUTION
Inadequate protein	Protein, p. 7, 8; Brewer's yeast, pages 45, 47
Poor-quality food or unbalanced diet	Food, p. 10, 22, 40, 41
Needs additional nutrients	Supplementation, pages 39–44
Poor absorption of nutrients	Vegetable enzymes, p. 145

UNHEALTHY PADS (CRACKED, HARD) (SEE UNHEALTHY WHISKERS)

VOMITING

POSSIBLE DIET PROBLEM	SOLUTION
Rancid/spoiled food	Canned food, page 19
Eating fatty foods/garbage	Not allowing it
Eating grass/plants	Fiber, pages 9, 10
Eating too fast	Mealtime mistakes, pages 28, 31
Overeating	Mealtime mistakes, p. 32
Intestinal problems	Intestinal problems; Acidophilus, p. 137 Digestive enzymes, p. 145
Gas	Excessive Gas, p. 53

INDEX